Antiprotozoal Drug Discovery: A Challenge That Remains

Edited By

Norma Rivera
Laboratory of Malariology
Department of Microbiology and Parasitology
Faculty of Medicine
UNAM
Mexico

Bentham Science Publishers Ltd.
Executive Suite Y - 2
PO Box 7917, Saif Zone
Sharjah, U.A.E.
Email: subscriptions@benthamscience.org

BENTHAM SCIENCE

CONTENTS

FOREWORD

All living creatures have to adjust to the cycle of life. All species have a beginning and have an end and during this period, they experience a breakdown of the homeostasis, call disease. Disease in man is associated to pain, anguish and suffering of the sick individual. More than a million years have been expended to search the causes of diseases, their effects in the body, and how to return patients to health. So many treatment procedures have emerged through human history, from natural products and magic healers to synthetic drugs design and physicians. As you can see, the application of curative measures have not frontiers nor limits.

Probably plants have been the principal source of remedies against disease. Actually, the use of plants, is not very practiced in occidental official medicine, instead, drugs are synthetic compounds that were primarily isolated from plants, fungus, algae, or bacteria. Nowadays, pharmacological industries, make big investments to develop new compounds for chronic and degenerative diseases, but it seems that investment on research to develop new drugs for diseases of the poor, is not one of their goals.

This book approaches the different facets of some of the most important diseases produced by protozoan parasites, under the analysis of epidemiological facts, economical and social impact, prevention and control problems. An analysis of the studies on new drugs for protozoan parasitic diseases, their hopes and achievements, is offered. An overview of the use of medical plants to treat specifically Malaria and Chagas disease, is also presented, as well as the experimental results obtained with the application of various metals in the treatment of malaria, leishmaniasis, toxoplasmosis and trichomoniasis.

This book will be of interest to parasitologists, pharmacologists and chemists and those involved or interested in the isolation and synthesis of active compounds against parasites.

Filiberto Malagón
Laboratory of Malariology
Department of Microbiology and Parasitology
Faculty of Medicine
UNAM
Mexico

PREFACE

Protozoan parasites are a worldwide public health problem that challenge the immune system of millions of humans and non-humans animals, resulting in devastating social and economic consequences. Until now, chemotherapy is central to the control of most of the infections caused by these parasites in both medical and veterinary practice. Chemotherapy control, has been mainly compromised by the development of parasite drug resistance, drugs severe side-effects and toxicity, low to medium efficacy, high cost drugs, and the introduction of counterfeit drugs that are a threat to public health with many overwhelming effects for patients; consequently, the search for new antiprotozoal drugs is an urgent need.

The development of new drugs against these parasites, has been largely neglected because they mainly affect people living in extreme poverty with limited or non-marketing possibilities; for these reasons, in some endemic countries, herbal medicine has become an important and sustainable source of control.

This eBook is an effort of researches who work in the field of antiparasitic experimental chemotherapy and medical parasitology and it summarizes the progresses made in the field of chemotherapy and drug research against protozoan diseases. Synthetic and natural treatments to control Chagas disease, malaria, toxoplasmosis and other parasitic diseases, are discussed in order to open the possibility for applying these scientific progress in the field of antiprotozoal chemotherapy.

The editor and the authors would like to thank Bentham Science Publishers for providing the opportunity to bring this knowledge to the scientific community and to the general public.

Norma Rivera
Laboratory of Malariology
Department of Microbiology and Parasitology
Faculty of Medicine
UNAM
Mexico

List of Contributors

A. Valeria Pozzoli	LabMOr-INTECIN, Departamento de Química de la Facultad de Ingeniería, de la Universidad de Buenos Aires, Ciudad Autónoma de Buenos Aires, Argentina
Elba Carrasco	Laboratory of Malariology, Department of Microbiology and Parasitology, Faculty of Medicine, National Autonomous University of Mexico (UNAM), Mexico City, 04510, Mexico
Emmanuelle Alvarado-Alvarez	Centre for Science and Technology Studies 14, Luis Enrique Erro, National Polytechnic Institute, Michoacana, Venustiano Carranza, AP. 15240, Mexico City, Mexico
Filiberto Malagón	Laboratory of Malariology, Department of Microbiology and Parasitology, Faculty of Medicine, National Autonomous University of Mexico (UNAM), Mexico City, 04510, Mexico
Gloria Rojas	Laboratorio de Biología de Parásitos, Departamento de Microbiología y Parasitología, Facultad de Medicina, Universidad Nacional Autónoma de México, México City, 04510, México
Gumaro Cano-Gutierrez	School of Health Sciences, UVM, Campus Sur, Mexico City, Mexico
Luz Eugenia Alcántara-Quintana	Potosino Institute for Scientific Research, Road to San José Dam 4th 2055. AP. 78216, San Luis Potosí, Mexico
Larry A. Walker	National Center for Natural Products Research , University of Mississippi, University MS, 38677, USA Department of BioMolecular Sciences, Research Institute of Pharmaceutical Sciences, University of Mississippi, University MS, 38677, USA
Luis F. Montaño	Department of Cellular and Tissue Biology, Faculty of Medicine, National Autonomous University of Mexico, Mexico City, 04510, Mexico
Margarita Cabrera	Laboratorio de Biología de Parásitos, Departamento de Microbiología y Parasitología, Facultad de Medicina, Universidad Nacional Autónoma de México, México City, 04510, México
Marcela Rojas-Lemus	Department of Cellular and Tissue Biology, Faculty of Medicine, National Autonomous University of Mexico, Mexico City, 04510, Mexico
Martha Bucio	Laboratorio de Biología de Parásitos, Departamento de Microbiología y Parasitología, Facultad de Medicina, Universidad Nacional Autónoma de México, México City, 04510, México
Miriam A. Martins Alho	LabMOr-INTECIN, Departamento de Química de la Facultad de Ingeniería, de la Universidad de Buenos Aires, Ciudad Autónoma de Buenos Aires, Argentina

Mónica Salas-Rojas	National Medical Center, XXI Century, Mexican Social Security Institute. Doctores 330, Cuauhtémoc, AP. 06725, Mexico City
Norma Rivera	Laboratory of Malariology, Department of Microbiology and Parasitology, Faculty of Medicine, National Autonomous University of Mexico, Mexico City, 04510, Mexico
Paz M. Salazar Schettino	Laboratorio de Biología de Parásitos, Departamento de Microbiología y Parasitología, Facultad de Medicina, Universidad Nacional Autónoma de México, México City, 04510, México
Pius S. Fasinu	National Center for Natural Products Research , University of Mississippi, University MS, 38677, USA
Teresa I. Fortoul	Department of Cellular and Tissue Biology, Faculty of Medicine, National Autonomous University of Mexico, Mexico City, 04510, Mexico

Antiprotozoal Drug Discovery: A Challenge That Remains

CHAPTER 1

Protozoal Diseases: Importance and Prophylaxis

Filiberto Malagón* and **Elba Carrasco**

Laboratory of Malariology, Department of Microbiology and Parasitology, Faculty of Medicine, National Autonomous University of Mexico (UNAM), Mexico City, 04510, Mexico

Abstract: This chapter focuses on the effect that five parasitic diseases, produced by five protozoa, have on human health, namely: malaria, toxoplasmosis, Chagas disease, leishmaniasis and trichomoniasis. Our approach is the following: An analysis of the epidemiological components of these diseases in the context of the parasite's life cycle; an analysis of the modifications in the natural history of these diseases introduced by human activities such as: migration, iatrogenesis and increased human mobility due to technological advances in the transportation of merchandise and persons; an analysis of how immune suppression produced by other living agents and chemotherapy affects these diseases, and their dispersion by tissue grafts; an analysis of the impact that these diseases have on the society, communities and family economies of countries affected by them, as well as what is being done to prevent them. In conclusion we find that research on new drugs is absolutely necessary to alleviate suffering, but given that these diseases are inextricably linked to poverty, we have to think of poverty as a disease, and as such we have an obligation to prevent it and eradicate it, as in the many other diseases and ills that befall mankind.

Keywords: Chagas disease, Chemotherapy, Leishmaniasis, Malaria, New drugs, Parasitic diseases, Poverty, Prohylaxis, Protozoa, Toxoplasmosis, Trichomoniasis.

INTRODUCTION

The simplest forms of life among the eukaryote are the protozoa, just formed by one cell. The first protozoa probably evolved from the fusion of two bacteria 1.45 to 2.5 billion years ago [1]. These primogenital protozoa, diversified, organized,

* **Corresponding author Filiberto Malagón:** Laboratory of Malariology, Department of Microbiology and Parasitology, Faculty of Medicine, National Autonomous University of Mexico (UNAM), Mexico City, 04510, Mexico; Tel: 55 56232465; Fax: 55 56232386; E-mail: malagon@unam.mx

Norma Rivera (Ed.)

and evolved into multicellular creatures from the trilobites to man. When studding protozoan parasites of man, I suggest not to lose the perception that we, humans, descend from those primogenital protozoa. If we think of humans in this fashion, it is not difficult to recognize that when the cells that conform us face a pathogen protozoa they initiate a relation or confrontation eukaryote to eukaryote and if the balance favors the host the infection is eradicated, but if it favors the parasite, the infection is established [2]. However, in this interaction both may come to an understanding, *i.e.* if the parasite doesn't behave as a parasite then the host will tolerate it. This mutual acceptance is possibly the most common.

Of all the protozoa in nature a minuscule number have learned to use humans as substrate, and of all these, only five are discussed in this book because they are of special significance to human health. The five protozoa referred to in this chapter are: *Plasmodium spp.*, *Toxoplasma gondii*, *Trypanosoma cruzi*, *Leishmania* spp. and *Trichomonas vaginalis*. We will systematically discuss each one of these parasites in the following chapters. In this first chapter we will have a general discussion about all five regarding issues which we find of particular relevance to better understand their importance. The reader will find that in some sections the five parasites are addressed together, while in others we will deal with one parasite or disease specifically.

ECONOMIC IMPORTANCE

When we talk about the economic importance of a disease, we normally talk about the burden that the disease creates at a local, national or global level. Most measurements take into account the premature mortality, morbidity, impairment and disability caused by the disease in study. The study of the global burden of diseases has developed a tool to quantify and compare health between populations, using a joint measure of both mortality and disability called disability-adjusted life year or DALY that measures the loss expressed in years of life due to death or disability caused by a disease [3, 4]. There are however other values that can also give us an idea of the burden produced by a disease.

A general rule created by Sachs and Malaney states that where malaria prospers more, human societies will prosper less. There is an unmistakable correlation between malaria and poverty. A comparison between the gross domestic product (GDP) of malarial and non malarial countries of similar development showed a GDP of US$1,526 for the malarial countries while in the non malarial countries it was US$8,268. This represents a five-fold difference between the two, which suggests that malaria exerts a considerable pressure on the economic development of populations. In a study of the rate of economic growth over a period of 25 years (1965-1990), countries with large populations living in areas of high malarial transmission were compared with countries of similar socioeconomic status but with a lower rate of malaria transmission. The results showed that the former countries had an annual per capita growth of 0.4% while for the latter it was 2.3%. [5].

In a study examining the burden of neglected tropical diseases within the framework of the global burden of disease, malaria was listed as the 9th cause of human death at global level, with 39 million DALYs, and held 1st place in the mortality burden among the tropical diseases of the world in the year 2002 [3].

An analysis of malarial deaths in the sub-Saharan region of Africa, made in 2010, showed a mortality between 655,000 and 1.24 million, with an estimated 82.69 million years lost by disability and death (DALYs), and an associated economic cost of 5.8% of the total GDP of the African Sub-Saharan region. Very important improvements have been achieved in the control of malaria in this region, with the use of residual insecticides impregnated in bed-nets and sprayed in houses, in conjunction with the artemisinin-based combination therapy. However, *Anopheles* resistance to the four classes of insecticides used has been documented, including pyrethroids, the only insecticides used to impregnate bed-nets; the resistance of *P. falciparum* to artemisinin has also been documented [6].

Among human infections caused by parasites, toxoplasmosis is one of the more prevalent, affecting 30 to 50% of the human population. Despite the fact that the infection is long-lived, the vast majority of people remain asymptomatic. The lowest prevalence of toxoplasmosis, of about 1% occurs in some countries in the Far East, and the highest rates, above 90% are found in European and South-American countries. A study of ocular toxoplasmosis in 1042 patients in Southern Brazil showed a prevalence 30 times higher than in any other part of the world

[7]. While in another study on toxoplasmosis in 70,123 individuals from different parts of Mexico, conducted by Galvan-Ramirez from 1951 to 2012, a prevalence of 28.9% was found [8].

In the Netherlands, Kortbeek and colleagues detected 2 cases of infection by *T. gondii* per 10000 live births, and they calculated that 388 children were born infected nationally in 2006, which puts an estimated *Toxoplasma* burden at 2,300 DALYs [9]. In another study performed in the same country in 2009 to calculate the burden produced by 14 foodborne pathogens, Havelaar and colleagues concluded that in conjunction, they created a total burden of 13,500 DALYs and that *T. gondii* was the most important parasite of this group [10].

We think it of interest to note that some studies have found a correlation between latent asymptomatic toxoplasma infections and the development of several diseases, suggesting the existence of cause and effect between those latent infections and the development of cancer and other diseases [11]. In fact, some observations made in France statistically correlate an association between *T. gondii* infections and the development of malignant brain tumors, mainly in males, observations that suggest the need to research the existence of these processes in individual patients [12].

American trypanosomiasis exists in its natural form in the American Continent, from Texas in USA to Patagonia in Argentina. However, it is not limited to this continent. One of the effects of globalization has been the spread of Chagas disease to all continents due to people travelling from endemic countries, some of them manifesting late face cardiomyopathy of chronic infections, even after 30 years of residence in the host countries [13]. 1 to 1000 cases of Chagas disease have been detected in eleven countries in Europe; In Canada, five European countries, Australia and Japan, 1000 to 10,000 cases have been found; In Spain and 8 countries of Central and South America 10,000 to 100,000 cases have been detected; In USA and 10 countries from Central and South America, 100,000 to one million cases are found; and in Argentina, Brazil and Mexico more than one million cases occur [14].

The annual cost per person to treat Chagas diseases is of US$4,660, the per person lifelong expense of US$27,684, and the annual global cost of US$7.19 billion and of $188.80 billion for lifelong expenses of the total Chagas disease patients [15]. In the global mortality burden of tropical diseases in the world measure in 2002, Chagas disease occupied the place 18th among the most important tropical neglected diseases, with a DALYs of 667,000 [3].

Leishmaniasis is an underreported disease because it has to be notified only in 33 out of the 88 endemic countries; in many of these countries, leishmaniasis is treated by non-governmental organizations or by the private sector. In Sudan, Africa, it is estimated that 91% of all deaths for kala-azar are not registered, and in India as much as 20% of the extremely poor patients infected with *L. donovani* died with no diagnosis. Leishmaniasis epidemics are associated with wars, ecologic disasters, famine and forced migration. During the civil war in Sudan, Africa, hundreds of thousands of visceral leishmaniasis cases occurred, in some communities causing the death of between 30 to 60% of the population. Possibly the first visceral epidemics occurred in Bengal and Assam in India where a devastating epidemic of a febrile chronic disease with cachexia, hepato-splenomegaly and a high fatality was described. Visceral leishmaniasis produced in South Asia (India, Nepal, Bangladesh) accounts for 60% of the global incidence. The cost of health care for kala-azar patients in these countries goes from US$80 to US$120, this equals or surpasses the annual per capita income of the patients and their families, aggravated by their inability to work and the frequent appearance of post-kala-azar dermal leishmaniasis.

In the Americas, Brazil suffers from 90% of visceral leishmaniasis cases and is regarded as the third most important concentration of visceral leishmaniasis in the world. Kala-azar from endemic countries of South Asia, differs from those of the Americas in that the first is produced by *L. donovani* and is transmitted only among humans, while the latter is produced by *L. chagasi* (*infantum*) and has a zoonotic character, in which dogs play the role of reservoirs. Infection occurs in rural, periurban and urban areas, marked by poverty. The cost of treatment with pentavalent antimony for a person is approximately of US$345. Brazil paid the equivalent of US$2.5 million in the treatment of 35,000 persons, plus $500,000 in the treatment of 95 persons with liposomal amphotericin [16, 17]. In 2002, leishmaniasis occupied the 9th place in mortality rate among the tropical diseases of the world, with 2,090,000 DALYs [3].

Trichomoniasis is the most prevalent sexually transmitted infection. It is estimated that in the USA 3% of the population is infected with *Trichomonas vaginalis*, with a proportionally higher rate in blacks than whites. Each year, it is calculated that 1.1 million new cases occur. Trichomoniasis is considered a neglected parasitic infection, perhaps because 70 to 85% of infected individuals do not develop symptoms, the infection is curable, and the general public lacks an interest in this disease [18]. Trichomoniasis is the last on the list of lifelong costs for direct medical care of 8 sexually transmitted infections, because it costs the US Government only 24 million dollars per year [19]. However, it is thought by some that trichomoniasis should be given more importance in the USA, because vaginal trichomoniasis in women can increase the risk of adverse effects during pregnancy including preterm delivery and low-birth-weight infants. Some observations also suggest that trichomoniasis in women increases their risk of acquiring HIV. In men trichomoniasis can cause urethritis complicated with prostatitis. These facts suggest that it would be wise to include trichomoniasis among reportable diseases in the USA [20].

EPIDEMIOLOGICAL IMPORTANCE

The Parasite Reservoir of Infection

From the five diseases discussed in this chapter, Chagas disease, leishmaniasis and toxoplasmosis have sylvatic or domestic animals other than man as parasite source of the infection, for which these are consider zoonosis, although, under certain circumstances humans may function also as source of parasites [21, 22, 23]. From the parasites causing these three diseases, *T. gondii* is the most widely disperse among different animal species (eurixenous) followed by *T. cruzi*, and *Leishmania* spp.

Malaria is produced by five parasite species: *P. falciparum*, *P. vivax*, *P. malariae* and *P. ovale* and *P. knowlesi* that causes malaria in macaques and humans in Southeast Asia [24]. In malaria knowlesi, Anopheles mosquitos use monkeys as the main source of the parasite to transmit the infection among other monkeys and humans, thus malaria also qualifies as a zoonosis, at least for this *Plasmodium* species. It is necessary to note that malaria parasites are also widely dispersed in nature in reptiles, birds and mammals, however, it differs from *Toxoplasma* because the same species of this parasite infects all its species of hosts, while the malaria parasite species are almost strictly specific for a host species [25]. Trichomoniasis is the only disease of the five that has the same animal species, *Homo sapiens*, as main host and reservoir. Due to its character as a sexually transmitted disease, trichomoniasis infections occurs only among humans, and both men and women may function as reservoir and transmitters.

Processes of Parasite Dispersion

A parasite is regarded as stenoxenous when it infects just one specie of host in nature; however, when a parasite is capable of infecting many host species, we regard it as eurixenous. A parasite that requires a single host to develop its complete life cycle is called a monoxenous parasite, and if it requires of more than one host to complete its life cycle is named polixenous. In a polixenous parasite, the species that hosts the sexual form of the parasite is called the definitive host, and the one that hosts the asexual form is called the intermediary host. The survival success of a parasite, relies on its capacity of dispersion in as many different host species and ecosystems as possible. The mechanisms of dispersion used among parasites, can be seen as different evolutionary processes developed by the parasite to adapt to the internal medium of their hosts, as well as to the external environment where it thrives.

To ensure dispersal, most parasites must leave their host to complete another part of their lifecycle. By leaving the host and entering the environment they develop infective forms that eventually reach a new host, however, some others have to enter another host, usually a blood sucking insect, in which the parasite produces its infective forms which are then transmitted by the insect to the new mammal host. Still others, use the host as definitive and intermediary host, *i.e.* they are parasites that develop the infective form in the same definitive mammal host.

Among the five parasitic protozoa under discussion, only *Toxoplasma gondii* leaves its host to continue its lifecycle in the environment through a resistant form, the oocyst, which is expelled in the feces of its definitive host, and exposed to aggressive environmental conditions such as chemical compounds in soil and water, changes in temperature, pH, humidity, nutrients, solar radiation, and predators. Some of these elements act as stimuli that prompt the metabolic changes required for differentiation and growth. With this parasite however we must take into account that the inactive forms (cysts) that develop in the tissues of its intermediary hosts are infective when eaten by other animal. This characteristic affords the parasite the greatest potential for dispersal possible as it introduces the parasite into the food chain. Other mechanisms are discussed below.

None of the other four parasites has a developmental stage which occurs outside its host. However, three out of the four, *Plasmodium* spp, *Trypanosoma cruzi* and *Leishmania* spp require a blood sucking insect that takes the parasite up when having a blood meal from the infected host allowing the parasite to complete its life cycle, producing in the interim, the infective forms that are dispersed when the insect takes another blood meal, now from the new host. However, the internal environment of these insects is so different from that of its vertebrate host in terms of nutrients, pH, temperature, ionic concentration, and cellular and chemical composition, that it exerts forces similar to those of the external environment, triggering metabolic changes that result in the differentiation of infective forms that makes dispersion in other vertebrate hosts.

Trichomonas vaginalis on the other side, does not require of any differentiation process or change to become infective and disperse in new hosts, it is not exposed to external environment conditions, this could explain the absence of resistant forms in this parasite. *T. vaginalis*, does not need of any other host species to disperse. As the parasite establishes itself in the sexual organs of its host, it uses its host's reproductive process to disperse from one individual to another during intercourse between females and males of the same species. Although occasionally this parasite can be transferred from one individual to another through fomites where it can survive for a short time.

Ingress of Parasite to Host

Protozoan parasites generally enter their hosts through the skin, mouth, nose, conjunctiva, placenta and sexual organs. Once they are inside, some species remain in the site of entrance, and get established there, while others migrate to some organ or tissue where they establish. On the whole, there is almost no tissue, organ or system in the body free of at least one kind of parasite, helminth or protozoa.

Mechanisms of Transmission

T. gondii is a totally eurixenous parasite that infects almost all warm-blooded animals, with no distinction of species. Man is number one predator in nature and there are almost no animal species unpalatable to him. This fact probably creates a higher risk of infection in humans by this parasite. All stages in the life cycle of *T. gondii* are potentially infective, irrespective of the animal species that play the role of reservoir. This Apicomplexan parasite possesses wide and varied mechanisms of transmission which may include the following: drinking water and eating food contaminated with oocysts, eating raw meat infected with cysts, by transfusion, by lactation, through the placenta during gestation, by organ grafts, eating uncooked eggs, or by passing through skin lesions.

Malaria, Chagas disease and leishmaniasis are diseases transmitted among their mammal, bird and reptile hosts, by hematophagous insects: anopheline mosquitoes in malaria, kissing bugs in Chagas disease and sandflies in leishmaniasis. The presence of these insects and the species required in each case is what causes the presence or absence of the disease. The fact that these diseases are transmitted by insects, has high epidemiological implications, because transmission of these diseases to humans is affected by all factors that regulate the insect population namely: environmental temperature, rain and lack thereof, winds, humidity, altitude above sea level, time of day of activity, flight range, natural refuges and blood sucking preferences. All these factors taken together may explain the vector potential of the insects and the geographical distribution of vectors and diseases.

From the vector viewpoint, malaria is a disease controlled by the presence of anopheline mosquitoes which can be found everywhere on earth; in regions where malaria is both endemic and non endemic, in temperate, tropical and periartic climate. However, the development of malaria parasites in the mosquito is dependent on temperature and the parasite can only continue its life cycle if the temperature of the mosquito is above 16ºC. As mosquitoes and arthropods in general do not posses mechanisms to control their body temperature, the mosquito's internal temperature will be the same as the ambient temperature where it lives, thus mosquitoes that live in areas where summer isotherms are below 16ºC will never become infected, and malaria transmission at these latitudes is not possible. This explains why the distribution of malaria is confined mainly to the tropics and to a lesser extent, subtropic and temperate climates. Another necessary factor is the presence of bodies of water large enough for the mosquitoes to breed in.

Some of the Central and South Pacific Islands are an example of regions with all the climatic and environmental conditions for the malaria to thrive, but where malaria had been absent, because no anopheles mosquitoes existed there. However, during the Second World War, warships introduced anopheles mosquitoes to some of these islands, where malaria transmission occurred later for some time [26]. Considering that the ability of the malaria parasite to grow in its insect host is temperature dependent, the global rise of temperature is a latent menace on the potential amplification of the geographic limits of malaria transmission on the planet.

Chagas disease occurs in its natural form only in the American Continent, because the kissing bug, exists only in this continent. The principal bug genera involved in transmission are: *Triatoma*, *Rhodnius*, and *Panstrongylus*. The infective forms are present in the bug´s feces and they are not released through the proboscis when biting, they are deposited on the skin during the bite and will enter the skin through the wound left by the bite, or carried to the conjunctiva mucous membranes. Sometimes Chagas disease transmission occurs orally when drinking beverages or eating food is contaminated with the bug's excrements. In these cases, in absence of the vector, this oral transmission of *T. cruzi* may produce micro epidemics as has been observed in Brazil, Colombia, and Venezuela [27]. In Mexico the distribution of the kissing bugs is limited by altitude and thus the infection and transmission occurs in areas located below 1,200 MSL.

All species of *Leishmania* both dermotropic and viscerotropic are transmitted through the biting of a blood sucking insect of the genus *Phlebotomus* (sandflies) in the Old World, and *Lutzomyia* in the New World. In the Old World there are two viscerotropic species of *Leishmania* with different behavior, *L. infantum* located in the Mediterranean that produces zoonotic infections in dogs and humans. Sandflies get the parasite from dogs or humans and return the parasite in its infective forms to humans and dogs. In South Asia, however, where three countries produce 60% of the visceral leishmaniasis of the world, the parasite species involved is *L. donovani* which produces infections among humans with no animal reservoirs.

In the New World, Brazil is the country that produces 90% of visceral leishmaniasis in the American Continent. In this country *L. chagasi*, a parasite related to *L. infantum*, is transmitted by *L. longipalpis*, and behaves like a zoonosis with the dog as animal reservoir, with the addition in this case of sylvatic foxes and opossums. In Brazil, Kala-azar is a sylvatic disease, however, since 1980 some of the biggest cities have seen an urbanization of the disease [28, 29].

Trichomonas vaginalis is a parasite with a one stage life cycle. The trophozoite lacks resistant forms to survive outside its hosts and has no transmission by vectors. Changes in environmental conditions do not exert any influence on the development of the parasite, or in its transmission, unless changes of the environment affect sexual activity or sexual behavior.

Congenital Transmission

Among our five parasites in discussion those classically involved in congenital infections are, without doubt, *Toxoplasma gondii* and *Plasmodium* spp. followed by *Trypanosoma cruzi* and *Leishmania donovani* [30].

An annual global incidence of 190,100 cases of congenital toxoplasmosis was estimated in 2008, equivalent to 1.2 million DALYs. The highest burdens were registered in South America and some other countries of low-income and middle East [31].

In *Plasmodium*, the species more involved in congenital transmission are *P. falciparum* and *P. vivax*. Studies of pregnant African women found that 24 million women were affected by malaria, and globally it is estimated that 75,000 to 200,000 unborn and newborn babies died from malaria, mostly in women suffering from asymptomatic malaria infections [32, 33].

In a study of Chagas disease cases in Brazil between 1980 and 2013 specifically regarding congenital transmission in pregnant women, it was found that of 549,359 pregnant women, 1,687 infected babies were born. It was found that the prevalence of Chagas disease among the women ranged from 0.1 to 8.5% according to the regions where they were attended and the congenital transmission rate was from 0% to 5.2%. The highest prevalence of *T. cruzi* infected pregnant women was found in the state of Bahia (4.65%) and Sao Paulo (2.9%). In 2010 the estimated number of Brazilian women of childbearing age was 683,217 and the expected number of pregnant women was of 34,629, of these, 589 women were expected to give birth to *T. cruzi* congenitally infected babies, producing an incidence of 18.7 congenital cases per 100,000 newborn babies [34].

Due to the fact that *T. cruzi* produces lifelong infections, women may perpetuate the infection by transmitting *T. cruzi* to their children through the placenta, which may be repeated in each pregnancy. This behavior gives the parasite a unique potential to perpetuate the infection (symptomatic or asymptomatic) in non endemic regions, from mother to child for an unknown number of generations without the need of a vector.

Congenital visceral leishmaniasis is very uncommon and most cases have been described in non endemic countries [35]. One case was described in Germany in which a 15 month old child, who had never left Germany, presented a classical clinical picture of visceral leishmaniasis, with no demonstration of leishmanial amastigotes in biopsies of liver and bone marrow, but with isolation of promastigotes in the cultures of his biopsies. His mother, completely asymptomatic was positive to titles of antibodies against antigens of the *L. donovani* complex, however, she had previously taken a trip to the Mediterranean, where she could have acquired a subclinical infection before pregnancy with no clinical signs of visceral leishmaniasis, and with no presence of the parasite in biopsies of liver, spleen and bone marrow. Since its first description by Low and Cook in 1926, until 1995, only seven cases of congenital visceral leishmaniasis had been published [30].

There are no congenital infections produced by *T. vaginalis*, however, the infection may in exceptional cases be passed to some newborn baby girls when going through the delivery channel of mothers with severe vaginal trichomoniasis [36].

Iatrogenic Transmission

By Transfusion

There are in the Americas more than 20 different countries with a wide spectrum of *T. cruzi* infected blood donors that range from 0.01 in USA to 60% in some Bolivian cities [37]. The procedures used by blood banks are never 100% safe, because a 2005 study in which the more sensitive techniques of blood screening were applied to detect *T. cruzi* in bank bloods, reported that there was still a residual risk of producing one case of transfusional Chagas for every 200,000 blood units applied in endemic zones [38].

Transfusional malaria is a problem for blood banks that stems from an unsatisfactory selection of blood donors, and the biggest problem for the banks is that donors show no signs of disease, even if they have stayed in areas of transmission. These asymptomatic donors could be infected with any species of *Plasmodium*, however, *P. malariae* is the most worrisome because this species produces the most benign clinical picture of malaria and the most asymptomatic patients [39].

Post transfusion malaria is, from many viewpoints a controversial subject which makes it a fascinating problem. Most countries located in hyperendemic areas (Sub-Saharian Africa), don't exclude malarious donors, because malaria is so widely disseminated in the region that if they rejected them there would be a drastic reduction in blood donations and therefore in transfusions. In any case, it is expected that those transfused patients will be exposed to malarial infection once they leave the hospital [40].

We have to remember that malaria parasites lyse the erythrocytes, and complicate the infection with severe anemia. This complication by *P. falciparum* is usually common in African children, of about 5 years old or less living in endemic areas, and these children require a blood transfusion as part of their treatment. In the Imo state University Hospital of Nigeria, an area where malaria is hyperendemic, it is considered appropriate to transfuse a patient when parasitemia reaches between 45 and 80%, *i.e.* transfusing patients that according to their standards have a median or high parasitemia, with a high decrease in hemoglobin concentration [41].

The issue of malarial blood from a donor being passed to a recipient who is also infected with malaria, leads us to the following reflections: Sub-Saharian Africa had 857 million inhabitants in 2010 who donated 4 million blood units each year. The major need for transfusions is linked to malaria infections. Children with severe malaria with less than 5g/L of hemoglobin, become eligible for transfusion, and is estimated that of all the individuals with confirmed cases of malaria, 5% will develop severe anemia, that would be 4,020,315 annual cases. If all these patients received a transfusion of just one unit of blood each, the total blood units collected in all Sub-Saharan Africa in a year would be exhausted [42].

Thinking about surgeries, obstetrical bleedings, accidents, and the many other medical situations that also require blood transfusions, the situation becomes alarming. However, many questions remain unanswered, one of them is what is the result of adding malaria parasites to a preexisting malaria infection? And who benefits, the parasite or the host?

Although in most countries of the developed world blood donors are very strictly vetted, in France, where 700 cases of post-transfusion malaria were reported annually until 2004, it is regarded as a minor problem, and they have a very relaxed donor selection system because in France, the experience has been that the post transfusion malaria risk is very small, to the order of 0.2 to 0.5 cases per million of blood units applied [43]. In malaria regions outside Africa, Venezuela for instance, it has been demonstrated that 0.8% of blood from donors residing in non-endemic areas shows anti-*P. falciparum* antibodies, while the blood coming from donors from endemic areas shows 3.8%, [44]. In most countries in Latin America, this *P. falciparum* positive blood would be discarded, because of its potential to produce post-transfusion malaria.

Due to the high number of individuals infected by *L. chagasi* (*infantum*) that remain asymptomatic, visceral leishmaniasis is a good candidate for post-transfusion transmission. In a study of 700 blood samples from blood banks in Bahia, Salvador, Brazil, to detect *L. chagasi* by means of the ELISA test, it was found that 38 (5.4%) of the samples were positive to antibodies against *Leishmania*, results that were found to be low, compared with other results observed in more endemic regions of visceral leishmaniasis in Brazil, such as the 9% reported in Natal and the 15.6% in Rio Grande do Sul. It is interesting to note that of the 38 positive samples, in the Bahia study, in 26 of them (68.4%) it was possible to prove the presence of *L. chagasi* by the detection of parasites DNA. Although the risk of transferring the infection with blood is real, no clinical symptoms seem to develop in the transfused individuals, and in Brazil leishmania testing in blood Banks is not mandatory [45].

Sicilia, Italy, reported a seropositivity of 0.75% to antigens of *L. infantum* in blood banks, from asymptomatic blood donors [46]. In Istanbul, Turkey, 0.5% of seropositive blood from 188 healthy individuals was detected in a blood bank, and in the Baleares islands in Spain 2.4% seropositivity was detected with ELISA in donor blood and 7.5% with Western blot [47, 48].

Ethiopia is a country of high HIV/AIDS endemicity with about 1.5 million individuals infected, of which between 5 to 7% live in or around Bahir Dar. A study on seroprevalence in the healthy blood donor population of Bahir Dar, measured by ELISA anti-*Toxoplasma* specific IgG and IgM antibodies showed a seropositivity of 70.29% (IgG), while individuals infected with HIV/AIDS exhibited anti-*Toxoplasma* antibodies in 87.4% (IgG) [49]. In another study done at the blood bank of the University Hospital of Imam Reza in Teheran, Iran, 122 cell packages and 101 fresh frozen plasma were submitted to detection of specific anti IgG-IgM anti-*Toxoplasma* antibodies, it was found that 49% of the cell packages were positive for IgG and 26% of fresh frozen plasma were positive to IgG anti-*Toxoplasma gondii* and just one of these samples was positive to IgM [50].

Transmission by Organ and Tissue Grafts

Parasite infections may be transferred from person to person in organ transplants. Two different situations may be observed in the recipients of organ grafts, in the first case, a seronegative recipient with no history of previous infection, becomes seropositive after the transplant, in this case the transplanted organ conveyed the parasite. In the second case, the recipient patient has an inactive infection and is therefore, seropositive before the transplant. After receiving an organ from a donor with no history of infection by the same parasite, the infection is clinically manifested, in this case, the recipient's old infection has revived due to the imposed immunosuppression after the transplant.

In Argentina 4.6% of organs from deceased donors were infected by *Trypanosoma cruzi* in 2009. Out of a waiting list of 7398 patients, 571 received transplants in Argentina in the first three months of 2013. In another study 26 Chagas seronegative organ recipients received an organ from seropositive donors, under strict monitoring for post-transplant infection, just one out of the 26 became infected, and received treatment [51].

In a study at the School of Medicine of Istanbul, Turkey, 106 Turkish patients that had received a non commercial live kidney transplant in India, 2 to 4 weeks previously were admitted to the hospital. Of the 106 patients, 10 developed post-transplant malaria complications [52]. Malaria complications in organ transplants is very uncommon in countries where malaria is not endemic if the donor is a resident of that country and has no history of malaria or travelling to foreign countries. When a post-transplant malaria complication is present, any species of *Plasmodium* may be involved. The most common cases of post-transplant malaria occur in kidney, heart, bone marrow and liver transplants [53, 54].

If one considers the high prevalence of individuals infected by *T. gondii*, and the fact that the vast majority of them remain infected but asymptomatic throughout their lifetime, is reasonable to assume that *Toxoplasma* is frequently present in post-transplant infections. Moreover, patients are subjected to immunosuppression as part of their treatment which may activate toxoplasma cysts that will eventually be present in the tissues of the receptor, or facilitate the activation of cysts present in the transplanted organ, as seem to be the case of the liver transplant described by Assi *et al.* in 2006 [55].

It is probable that about 3% of patients receiving a transplanted kidney in the University Hospital of Medical Science in Tehran, Iran, acquired a toxoplasmosis infection transferred by the transplanted organ [56]. In another case, a heart from a *Toxoplasma* seropositive donor (IgG) was transplanted to a seropositive recipient without anti-toxoplasma prophylactic medication, which resulted in a disseminated toxoplasmosis to lungs, liver, spleen, brain and heart [57]. In general it can be said that clinically manifested toxoplasmosis in post-transplanted patients may result in death, especially in seronegative *Toxoplasma* patients that receive a heart transplant from a seropositive donor [58].

With certain frequency visceral leishmaniasis is present as a complication in patients that receive an organ transplant, most commonly in kidney transplant, although, it has also been reported also in liver, heart, lung, pancreas and bone marrow transplants [59, 60]. Most of these recipient patients live or have travelled to endemic regions of kala-azar. Usually it is very difficult to distinguish when a post-transplant visceral leishmaniasis is due to the reactivation of an asymptomatic infection already present in the recipient, or if it was induced by parasites present in the transplanted organ, however, once the infection is established and treated successfully, several relapses may occur [61]. As a result of these relapses, some of these patients may develop cutaneous or mucocutaneous post-kala-azar complications, putting their life in danger [62].

Parasites and Immune-suppression

Individuals are immunosuppressed by the effects of chronic stress, pregnancy, immunosuppressive infections such as AIDS, the administration of immuno-suppressive medicines as therapy in autoimmune and rheumatological diseases, by transplants of solid organs and stem cells and chemotherapy and therapeutic radiations for treatment of cancer. Immunosuppression produces a high susceptibility and vulnerability to any kind of infection. Patients infected with HIV could receive a superimposed infection by any of our five protozoa, with potentially dramatic results. In the Mediterranean region of Europe, visceral leishmaniasis is the third most frequent opportunistic infection among HIV positive patients, and may become fatal in some cases, while cutaneous leishmaniasis may transform into diffused cutaneous leishmaniasis or be disseminated to the reticuloendothelial system and other organs. Both types of leishmaniasis frequently produce relapses after treatment [63, 64].

When *T. gondii* functions as an opportunist parasite aggregated to immuno-compromised patients, it can invade central nervous system with clinical manifestations of encephalitis that may be terminal [65]. Cohelo and colleagues, made a 25 years review study on opportunistic infections in 3378 AIDS patients who attended the Fio Cruz Institute in Rio de Janeiro, Brazil, and showed that cerebral toxoplasmosis occupied the third place among opportunistic infections just after tuberculosis and esophagic candidiasis [66].

In malaria, however, a clear negative correlation that favors malaria or HIV infections has not been found. Some authors state that malaria is less associated with HIV immunosuppression than other opportunistic infections [67], while others don't find that immunosuppression by the virus worsens a malaria infection, don't mention if it modifies the course of the viral infection in any way. This situation is explicable in part by the fact that the antimalarial treatment has a certain antiviral effect, and the anti-retroviral exhibits a certain antimalarial effect, as demonstrated by assays with mefloquine that were found to be active against HIV and malaria. It isn't known, however, if any synergies result if simultaneous treatments are given [68].

In other situation, a subject primarily infected with any of our five protozoa or any other infectious agent, is secondarily infected with HIV. In this case, the state of immunosuppression caused by the virus, may have a reactivating effect on undetermined phase of chronic Chagas disease [69], on unapparent infections by *T. gondii* and *Leishmania* species, although in the case of malaria infections it seems not to have any effect, as above commented.

Infections by *T. vaginalis* augment susceptibility to infections by bacteria and HIV. This seems to occur due to the changes produced by the parasite on vaginal microbiota, causing an increase of pH, and damage to the vaginal epithelium that favors the entrance of HIV [70].

The Movement of Parasites Worldwide

Since his origin millions of years ago, man has been in constant movement, following and finding his food, slowly occupying all the ecosystems of the earth, from jungles to deserts. Domestication of plants and animals brought about a sedentary life and the formation and organization of communities, towns and cities, however it does not put an end to human mobilization. This movement by foot, horse, donkey, mule, camel and elephant, has been changed to railways, cars, ships and airplanes. Modern systems of transportation have made the world small, and every single place on earth is now accessible for exploring, trading, studying, working, or just visiting for the sheer pleasure of exploring places, cultures and people.

Humans do not escape to the laws of nature, and so they are preyed upon by other creatures, just as humans do. Mostly we humans are invaded by parasites of every kind (virus, bacteria, protozoan, and metazoan), which make no noise, they don't disturb us, they feed from us without provoking homeostatic imbalances, so usually we are unaware of these creatures living inside us. We move with them wherever we go, giving our parasites an opportunity to look for other human or animal hosts, *i.e.* we share our parasites with other animals. Therefore, when we return from our journeys we have left some of our parasites in the places we visited, and we have brought home some of the parasites we found in the lands we visited, without being aware of it most of the time.

In 2011, as many as 1110 million persons traveled by air and it is expected to increase to 1450 millions for 2016. Never in history have the malaria endemic zones been better connected with the rest of the world, which facilitate the movement of malaria and other diseases between endemic and non endemic regions [71].

It is common that migrants or tourists visiting malaria endemic lands will return to their non endemic countries with a malaria infection, where they may clinically manifest the disease, or remain asymptomatic, in which case they become a risk if they donate blood or organs. The countries that have the highest number of cases of imported malaria are USA, Great Britain, France, and Canada [72]. *Plasmodium species* have a geographical distribution that is more or less defined. Sometimes, a traveler will introduce a foreign species of parasites to the non endemic region of his country, as was the case recently of *P. ovale* imported to Central America, with the danger that it will then establish as an endemic species [73].

The first detection of malaria in persons living in the proximities of airports in non-endemic countries was done in 1969. These malaria infections are usually produced by *P. falciparum* in absence of local malaria transmission and/or anopheline mosquitoes. It is supposed that infected mosquitoes arrive with airplanes coming from, or with stop-overs in airports in malaria endemic countries in Africa and bite airport employees. Most of the 89 cases reported were detected in Europe, principally in the airports of France, Belgium, United Kingdom, Italy, Netherlands, Spain and Switzerland.

However, some cases have been observed in other countries outside Europe, most recently in Tunisia, an African Mediterranean country where malaria had been eradicated since 1979. These four *P. falciparum* infections occurred in persons with no history of blood transfusion, nor addiction to drugs, that had not travelled outside Tunisia, but all of them residing in the same district, 2 kilometers away from the international airport of Tunis. Certainly, the authors think that the infections were produced by the bites of mosquitoes arriving in the airplanes, but no evidence exists to prove this supposition. In fact, it was not suggested in the hypothesis of these cases that the European cases previously reported had been proven, and the question of how the parasites reached these persons, remains a mystery [74 - 79].

Cutaneous leishmaniasis is mostly acquired by adventurous travelers who stay a long time in hyperendemic zones of the South American rain forests, while popular Mediterranean destinations are the principal areas for tourists to acquire visceral leishmaniasis [80, 81]. People that arrive to Australia with leishmaniasis, show mostly the dermotropic type, with a history of traveling or living in Afghanistan [82].

Chagas disease is not known as a disease that travelers need to fear, because if they stay in standard accommodation in any part of Latin America, there is no risk of acquiring the infection. However, if travelers stay in small towns far from urban areas, in dwellings with traditional roof and wall materials, the risk of a kissing bug infestation is present and thus the possibility of *T. cruzi* transmission [83, 84]. Although, it has to be said that travelers that enjoy traditional food and beverages in South American countries are at risk a *T. cruzi* infection by oral route even in the absence of the kissing bugs [27].

Toxoplasmosis is perhaps the most widespread parasitic disease, because *T. gondii* is the parasite species with the widest dispersion in nature. It infects most warm-blooded animals, with the development of infective tissue cysts in most of them, so the ingestion of raw or badly cooked meat of almost all birds and mammals carries the risk of a *T. gondii* infection. In Paris, France, a traveler is exposed to toxoplasmosis as any other resident of this city when eating European or imported horse meat [85]. 17% of French lamb meat and 89% of their sheep meat is infected by *T.gondii*, as is pork meat, regardless of its origin, national or imported [86, 87].

Trichomoniasis is a disease that travelers bring with them and they transmit and/or acquire the local strain when the journey's pleasures include sexual relations.

PROPHYLAXIS

The prophylaxis and measures to prevent protozoan diseases just as those caused by any other parasite, are dictated by the correct interpretation of their life cycle and the elements that regulate it, *i.e.* parasite, host and environment.

In Chagas disease *T. cruzi*, is dispersed from infected mother to her fetus or between vertebrate hosts with the help of the bite-defecation of the kissing bug, the urine of bats and opossum dejections feces, organ transplants or transfusions, entering the new host through the skin, mucous epithelium, and blood, depending on the parasite source. Ideally, in this case prevention would be achieved by eliminating the parasite in humans, animals and bugs. Since from a practical point of view it would be impossible to eliminate *T. cruzi* infections circulating between sylvatic animals and kissing bugs, sources of parasites for human infections will persist while the sylvatic cycle exists, thus the elimination of human infections is impossible [88].

Elimination of parasites is confined then to man-domicilary kissing bugs, people and domestic animals. In this context some problems arise, first, because vector species strictly domiciliary with man are few, most of them are species that live with man but maintain a sylvatic nexus [89]. This implies that if the domestic bugs were eliminated, they would be replaced by sylvatic ones of the same species. Secondly, we have to remember that once humans are infected by *T. cruzi* they are infected for life, and there is no highly successful medicine available to eliminate the tissue forms of the parasite. Chemotherapy certainly diminishes the parasite burden and brings a decrease in the transmissibility of the infection, but it doesn't eliminate all the parasites nor the possibility of infecting vectors [90].

Other problems are related to the resistance of the kissing bugs to insecticides, and parasites to drugs [91, 92]. Prevention of Chagas transmission by transfusion and organ transplants are very complex medical problems that are not limited to a good donor selection practice, because there are cases of asymptomatic infected donors, with no history of previous infection and with no way to diagnosis.

Prevention of Chagas disease acquired by oral route unfolds a new dimension of the disease connected to its urbanization. It has changed from a disease typically considered of a rural nature, becoming urban and with an absence of kissing bugs. In Venezuela, epidemic outbreaks due to oral transmission have occured in schools and families in urban and rural zones with unknown vectors, commonly associated with the ingestion of seasonal fruit juice [93]. General recommendations for diseases acquired by oral route, included to improved personal hygiene, protection of beverages and food, washing of fruits and vegetables *etc*.

Leishmaniasis endemic countries, the viscerotropic strain is a major concern. About 60% of the world visceral leishmaniasis occurs in the Indian subcontinent, where the poorest state of India, Bihar, produces the highest number of cases. WHO estimated an annual incidence for 2004-2008 from between 146,000 to 282,000 cases of visceral leishmaniasis and 10 to 20% did not receive treatment and died. In 2005, India, Nepal and Bangladesh signed an agreement to eliminate visceral leishmaniasis as a public health problem. The aim was to reach an incidence of one case per 10,000 inhabitants by spraying DDT in houses to eliminate *Phlebotomus argentipes*, the vector, and cure all patients with Amphotericin B, an old anti-mycotic now reformulated as liposomal amphotericin B applied in a single doses by intravenous route [94]. This was the last advance in a program that originally started using sodium stibogluconate, followed by miltefosine until 2010, when amphotericin B made its appearance.

In 2015, Lucero and colleagues gave us an account of his experience in Bangladesh in a 12 months post-treatment follow up of kala-azar patients: 3 out of 1179 patients died, 39 out of 1521 patients relapsed and 1479 patients out of 1521 were cured *i.e.* a fantastic 97%. In order to estimate the possible effect of this measure, one has to consider that no animal reservoirs of the infection other than man exists in India nor in Bangladesh [95], infection occurs man to man, by *L. donovani*.

Another component for the prevention of leishmanial infections is to avoid *Phlebotomus* and *Lutzomyia* biting, by the use of bednets and/or application of insecticides, DDT or the pyrethroids used nowadays. However, DDT is prohibited in many countries and is a pesticide that has produced resistance to vectors [96]. In India *Ph. argentipes* the principal vector, is resistant to DDT and susceptible to Malathion and the pyrethroid deltamethrin [97]. *Lutzomyia longipalpis* in America is still mostly susceptible to the most common insecticides.

As in other mosquito borne diseases, malaria prevention includes protection from mosquito biting and eliminating parasites from the blood of patients with antimalarial drugs. The 4-aminoquinoline, known as chloroquine, was the synthetic antimalarial drug that remained in general use since the World War II until 1957, when the first case of resistance to *P. falciparum* infection was detected in Thailand, confirmed two years later in Colombia and detected in Oriental Africa in 1970. At present, strains of *P. falciparum* resistant to chloroquine are spread all over the malarial world except Central America and Mexico where the parasite is still susceptible. Mefloquine substituted chloroquine in limited parts of the world for a short period of time, until artesunate finally substituted chloroquine, and has been in use as a basic antimalarial drug, later associated with other drugs to avoid the emergence of malaria parasite resistance, combinations that nowadays survive are the artesunate with: lumefantrine amodiaquine, mefloquine, sulfadoxine-pyrimethamine and dihydroartemisinin-piperaquine [98].

Poverty

Family income is determinant to ensure adequate food intake, housing, environmental health, education, clean living conditions, accessibility to health care services, habits, personal hygiene, *etc*.

Parasitic diseases are generally linked to poverty, and poverty is a chronic disease of people and countries all over the world those euphemistically known as "developing countries". In Latin America in 2012, the extremely poor added to the moderately poor made up 37% of the population [99].

In Latin America 15 to 17 million poor persons are infected with *T. cruzi* and another 90 to 100 million exposed to the infection [100]. Poverty, hunger and lack of employment have brought about big waves of human migration as consequence. People in movement from poor to developed countries go accompanied by their parasites. Eight years ago (2007) Schmunis [101], calculated that these migrant waves had included 103,718 individuals infected by *T. cruzi* that arrived only to Australia, Canada, Spain, and USA. In another study of Latin American migrants in Europe, Strasen and col. estimated in 2014 that there are in Europe more than 100,000 migrants infected by *T. cruzi* (including Spain), although 95% of them are not diagnosed [102].

Estimates in the USA indicated that in 2013 there were 300,000 cases of Chagas disease introduced by migrants coming from the endemic zones, and that 40,000 pregnant American women could be infected with *T. cruzi*, and of these pregnant women 2,000 cases of congenital Chagas may be expected [103]. These migrant receptor countries, except for the USA, don't have *T. cruzi* vectors, and are not endemic to Chagas disease, therefore, although the parasite has been introduced, natural transmission cannot be established. Their concern however, is the possibility that other mechanisms of transmission may occur such as transmission by transfusion, organ transplant, or congenital transmission.

Leishmaniasis is an endemic disease in 88 countries around the world with more than 350 million people at risk. In 2006 there was an estimated annual incidence of 2 million new cases, of which 0.5 million corresponded to visceral leishmaniasis and 1.5 million to dermal leishmaniasis. Visceral leishmaniasis produces 59,000 annual deaths, which cause 2,357,000 DALYs. Clinically for each one of the symptomatic cases of leismaniasis it is expected that there are 6 to 20 asymptomatic ones. Five countries, Bangladesh, Brazil, India, Nepal and Sudan, concentrate 90% of all visceral leishmaniasis cases in the world, and 90% of cutaneous leishmaniasis occur in Afghanistan, Algeria, Brazil, Iran, Peru, South Arabia and Sudan.

Leishmaniasis is present in countries with low development. India, a country of median income, has the major burden of visceral leishmaniasis in the world, and more than 90% of its cases are reported from Bihar the poorest Indian state [104]. Visceral leishmaniasis has been converted into an opportunistic infection in HIV/AIDS patients, contributing their risk of mortality [17].

In 2007 Vaginal trichomoniasis was present in 3.1% of American women of reproductive age (14-49 years old), however a racial disparity has been observed, because the prevalence in non Hispanic white women was of 1.3%, and 1.8% in Mexican American women while in black women was of 13.3%, that is as much as 10 times higher in this sector than in the other two. This study suggests poverty among other factors involved in the disparity. 512 black women between 14 to 18 years old in 2002, points out a series of risk factors that predispose a person to reinfections by *T. vaginalis*, all of them due to the environment of poverty in which these women grow up [105].

The clear and undeniable link of poverty and malaria has been discussed above. Exposure to toxoplasmosis may be different in wealthy, medium income and poor people, depending on the infective form of the parasite that infects the person. If the infection is started by oocysts, drinks or food contaminated with cat feces has to be ingested, which means a lack of general hygiene, bad quality of water, and an unsanitary environment, conditions that are linked to poverty.

If the infective form is the Bradizoite, it is present in the tissues of animal food (meat) and those who eat raw or badly cooked meat are at risk. The wealthy and medium income population eats more meat than the poor people, and thus they are more at risk, however, when poor people eat meat, if at all, it is probable that the meat will come from animals with no sanitary regulations, thus the risk is greater. In general, toxoplasmosis is more prevalent in tropical developing countries where the poor are abundant, however, in this context France would seem to be an exception, particularly in Paris, a wealthy community with about 90% of its population infected by *T. gondii*. In the United States, the official poverty rate in 2006 reached 12.3% of its population (according to their own poverty standards), which suffer of toxoplasmosis among other chronic and debilitating diseases known as neglected diseases of poverty [106].

In Latin America, as in the developing world, toxoplasmosis is also associated with poverty. In a study of seroprevalence to *T.gondii* performed on agricultural workers migrating internally from poor communities within the state of Durango, Mexico, the authors found a seroprevalence positive to *T. gondii* in 29% (IgG) of the workers, of which 20% were actively infected (IgM+) [107]. In a poor suburban community of Maracaibo, Venezuela, with a high population of cats, and a high annual new birth rate, Diaz-Suarez and Estevez in 2009 did a study on active infection of *T. gondii* measured by IgM anti-*Toxoplasma* antibodies in the women of childbearing age, finding a positive seroprevalence of 18.2% [108]. In a low income community called Jardim Sao Remo in the Municipality of Sao Paulo, Brazil a study of seroprevalence to *T. gondii* was done with indirect immunofluorescence, performed in children from 1 to 15 years old in 2002, the authors found 5.8% seropositivity in children between 1 and 3 years, and 56% in those between 13 to 15 years old. The earliest seroconversion was found in a 2 year old boy [109].

Poverty as Disease

Before concluding this last part of chapter I, I have to make clear, that if disease means the suffering of human beings and if the principal aim of a doctor is to eliminate the suffering of his or her patient; although the amelioration or elimination of suffering does not necessarily cure the disease, any effort to look for the best medicine to cure people of their diseases is the most noble action a human may undertake to alleviate suffering.

Drug discovery is always an attempt to reach this aim, but the following comments are a personal reflection on something we consider central to the real solution of parasitic diseases, and which we feel deserves to be shared with our readers.

A human being in poverty is in our opinion, a sick person whose sickness opens the door to other diseases. The daily stress of his or her misery afflicts the spirit and the immune system equally.

If we examine the diseases we are discussing as a whole, it may be noticed that the main element shared by all communities afflicted by these diseases is poverty. When discussing these diseases we're dealing with poor countries and poor communities. These are communities that suffer unimaginable deprivations in terms of education, food, housing, healthy environment, water for drinking and personal hygiene, medical services, minimal public health infrastructure, if any, *etc.*

Our response to the infectious diseases of these and all people has been to look for an effective drug to treat them, to look for a vaccine to prevent infections, to spread insecticides to kill the vectors, to give bed nets to avoid mosquito biting, and so on. In the best of cases some of these sick people get cured, but we have not solved the problem. Their poverty and all that it entails has not been changed, thus new infections or reinfections return, it becomes a vicious circle impossible to break while poverty persists.

If poverty and parasites are the problem, and if complete eradication of the parasites is not possible, we may try to eliminate poverty. To do this, however, we have to think differently, firstly we have to think of people as society's greatest asset, secondly, to think of every poor man as a sick man and thus of poverty as a disease, thirdly if poverty is a disease we have to study the burden of poverty, to see the effect of poverty on the progress of society and human kind, in the same way we now quantify the social burden of any of the diseases discussed.

In a world dominated by money and cost-benefit calculations, health and disease included, we have to be convinced that it is more beneficial to eradicate poverty than to perpetuate it. To start we have to ask ourselves how much does the burden of poverty disease cost society. If we performed this study, we would be able to quantify the disabilities and death that poverty causes and its lost value in DALYs. It is quite probable that the cost of poverty disease is higher than the individual, familiar, communal and national expenses caused by all the diseases that are associated with this central disease, poverty.

Perhaps the results of these studies would spur us to plan a global program to eradicate poverty disease. The eradication of poverty disease would have repercussions on many other diseases, which would benefit us all.

CONFLICT OF INTEREST

The authors confirm that they have no conflict of interest to declare for this publication.

ACKNOWLEDGEMENTS

The authors thank Project PAPIIT-DGAPA IN-229611, UNAM.

GLOSSARY

Amastigote	= A stage of *Trypanosome* and *Leishmania* parasites living in the tissue cells of their host.
Anopheline	= Related to the group of Anopheles mosquito, vector of the malaria parasites in mammals.
Apicomplexa	= Phylum that include protozoal parasites which have a group of organelles in their apex usually used for invading cells, like Coccidia, *Plasmodium, Cryptosporidium* and *Toxoplasma*, among many others.
Bradizoite	= An intracellular stage of *Toxoplasma gondii* characterized by slow rate of reproduction, and long survival in tissue of its host.
Dermotropic	= Preference of a parasite to localize in the skin.
Endemicity	= Denotes the presence of a disease regularly found in a defined region.
Esophagic	= Pertaining to the esophagus.
Eurixenous	= Parasites that infect many species of hosts.
Hematophagous	= used in Entomology to designate blood feeding arthropods.
Hyperendemic	= Refers to a disease, like malaria, with a high incidence in a defined area.

Iatrogenic	= Related to illness caused by medical management.
IgG, IgM	= Classes of immunoglobulins (antibodies) present in blood, and other body fluids.
Immunocompromised	= Refers to a person with an impaired immune system.
Kala-azar	= Another name for visceral leishmaniasis.
Lutzomyia	= Blood sucking insect vector of leishmaniasis in America.
Monoxenous	= Parasites that complete its life cycle in only one host species.
Mucocutaneous	= Parasitic lesions simultaneously found in skin and mucous membrane tissues.
Non-endemic	= Disease not regularly present in a geographically defined area.
Oocyst	= Stage of Apicomplexan parasites life cycle that house the infective form of the parasite, resistant to environmental conditions.
Parasitemia	= Defines the number of parasites that circulate in blood stream of a host.
Periarctic	= Around the Arctic Circle.
Promastigote	= The stage of *Trypanosome* and *Leishmania* parasites developing in the blood sucking insect vector.
Prophylaxis	= Applied to the actions taken to prevent a disease in an individual or a population
Polixenous	= Parasites that require more than one host species to complete its life cycle, a definitive host and one or more intermediary hosts.
Reticuloendothelial	= Tissue that forms the immune system.
Seroconversion	= Refers to a person or a population that has changed its condition from seronegative to seropositive in relation to the presence of antibodies against a parasite.
Seronegative	= That gives a negative result in a test of blood serum to detect a parasite.
Seropositivity	= That is in a state of positivity to test of blood serum to detect a parasite.
Seroprevalence	= The level of antibodies against a parasite present in the blood of a population.
Stenoxenous	= Parasite that infects a restricted number of host species.
Triatoma, Rhodnius, Panstrongylus	= Different genera of blood sucking bugs, vectors of Chagas disease, known as kissing bugs.
Trofozoite	= The trophic stage of protozoa.
Viscerotropic	= Preference of a parasite to localize in viscera.

REFERENCES

[1] Müller M, Mentel M, van Hellemond JJ, *et al.* Biochemistry and evolution of anaerobic energy metabolism in eukaryotes. Microbiol Mol Biol Rev 2012; 76(2): 444-95.
[PMID: 22688819]

[2] Barribeau SM, Sadd BM, du Plessis L, Schmid-Hempel P. Gene expression differences underlying genotype-by-genotype specificity in a host-parasite system. Proc Natl Acad Sci USA 2014; 111(9):

3496-501.
[PMID: 24550506]

[3] Mathers CD, Ezzati M, López AD. Measuring the burden of neglected tropical diseases: the global burden of disease framework. PLoS Negl Trop Dis 2007; 1(2): e114.
[PMID: 18060077]

[4] Murray CJ, Lopez AD. Evidence-based health policy--lessons from the Global Burden of Disease Study. Science 1996; 274(5288): 740-3.
[PMID: 8966556]

[5] Sachs J, Malaney P. The economic and social burden of malaria. Nature 2002; 415(6872): 680-5.
[PMID: 11832956]

[6] Tusting LS, Willey B, Lucas H, *et al.* Socioeconomic development as an intervention against malaria: a systematic review and meta-analysis. Lancet 2013; 382(9896): 963-72.
[PMID: 23790353]

[7] Glasner PD, Silveira C, Kruszon-Moran D, *et al.* An unusually high prevalence of ocular toxoplasmosis in southern Brazil. Am J Ophthalmol 1992; 114(2): 136-44.
[PMID: 1642287]

[8] Galvan-Ramirez MdeL, Troyo R, Roman S, Calvillo-Sanchez C, Bernal-Redondo R. A systematic review and meta-analysis of *Toxoplasma gondii* infection among the Mexican population. Parasit Vectors 2012; 5: 271.
[PMID: 23181616]

[9] Kortbeek LM, Hofhuis A, Nijhuis CD, Havelaar AH. Congenital toxoplasmosis and DALYs in the Netherlands. Mem Inst Oswaldo Cruz. Rio de 2009; 104: 370-3.

[10] Havelaar AH, Haagsma JA, Mangen MJ, *et al.* Disease burden of foodborne pathogens in the Netherlands, 2009. Int J Food Microbiol 2012; 156(3): 231-8.
[PMID: 22541392]

[11] Flegr J, Prandota J, Sovičková M, Israili ZH. Toxoplasmosis--a global threat. Correlation of latent toxoplasmosis with specific disease burden in a set of 88 countries. PLoS One 2014; 9(3): e90203.
[PMID: 24662942]

[12] Vittecoq M, Elguero E, Lafferty KD, *et al.* Brain cancer mortality rates increase with *Toxoplasma gondii* seroprevalence in France. Infect Genet Evol 2012; 12(2): 496-8.
[PMID: 22285308]

[13] Vannucchi V, Tomberli B, Zammarchi L, *et al.* Chagas disease as a cause of heart failure and ventricular arrhythmias in patients long removed from endemic areas: an emerging problem in Europe. J Cardiovasc Med 2014; 15: 1-7.

[14] Bonney KM. Chagas disease in the 21st century: a public health success or an emerging threat? Parasite 2014; 21: 11.
[PMID: 24626257]

[15] Lee BY, Bacon KM, Bottazzi ME, Hotez PJ. Global economic burden of Chagas disease: a computational simulation model. Lancet Infect Dis 2013; 13(4): 342-8.
[PMID: 23395248]

[16] Bern C, Maguire JH, Alvar J. Complexities of assessing the disease burden attributable to leishmaniasis. PLoS Negl Trop Dis 2008; 2(10): e313.
[PMID: 18958165]

[17] Reithinger R. Leishmaniases' burden of disease: ways forward for getting from speculation to reality. PLoS Negl Trop Dis 2008; 2(10): e285.
[PMID: 18958280]

[18] Meites E. Trichomoniasis: the "neglected" sexually transmitted disease. Infect Dis Clin North Am 2013; 27(4): 755-64.
[PMID: 24275268]

[19] Owusu-Edusei K Jr, Chesson HW, Gift TL, *et al.* The estimated direct medical cost of selected sexually transmitted infections in the United States, 2008. Sex Transm Dis 2013; 40(3): 197-201.
[PMID: 23403600]

[20] Hoots BE, Peterman TA, Torrone EA, Weinstock H, Meites E, Bolan GA. A Trich-y question: should *Trichomonas vaginalis* infection be reportable? Sex Transm Dis 2013; 40(2): 113-6.
[PMID: 23321992]

[21] Urdaneta-Morales S. Chagas' disease: an emergent urban zoonosis. The caracas valley (Venezuela) as an epidemiological model. Front Public Health 2014; 2: 265.
[PMID: 25520950]

[22] Roque AL, Jansen AM. Wild and synanthropic reservoirs of *Leishmania* species in the Americas. Int J Parasitol Parasites Wildl 2014; 3(3): 251-62.
[PMID: 25426421]

[23] Liu Q, Wang ZD, Huang SY, Zhu XQ. Diagnosis of toxoplasmosis and typing of *Toxoplasma gondii.* Parasit Vectors 2015; 8: 292.
[PMID: 26017718]

[24] Yusof R, Lau YL, Mahmud R, *et al.* High proportion of knowlesi malaria in recent malaria cases in Malaysia. Malar J 2014; 13: 168.
[PMID: 24886266]

[25] Garnham PC. Malaria Parasites and other haemosporidia. Oxford: Blackwell Scientific Publications 1966.

[26] Nowell WR. Vector introduction and malaria infection on Guam. J Am Mosq Control Assoc 1987; 3(2): 259-65.
[PMID: 3333056]

[27] Nóbrega AA, Garcia MH, Tatto E, *et al.* Oral transmission of Chagas disease by consumption of açaí palm fruit, Brazil. Emerg Infect Dis 2009; 15(4): 653-5.
[PMID: 19331764]

[28] Costa CH. Characterization and speculations on the urbanization of visceral leishmaniasis in Brazil. Cad. Saúde Pública. Rio de 2008; 24: 2959-63.

[29] Werneck GL, Costa CH, Walker AM, David JR, Wand M, Maguire JH. Multilevel modelling of the incidence of visceral leishmaniasis in Teresina, Brazil. Epidemiol Infect 2007; 135(2): 195-201.
[PMID: 16824254]

[30] Meinecke CK, Schottelius J, Oskam L, Fleischer B. Congenital transmission of visceral leishmaniasis (Kala Azar) from an asymptomatic mother to her child. Pediatrics 1999; 104(5): e65.
[PMID: 10545591]

[31] Torgerson PR, Mastroiacovo P. The global burden of congenital toxoplasmosis: a systematic review. Bull World Health Organ 2013; 91(7): 501-8.
[PMID: 23825877]

[32] Uneke CJ. Impact of placental *Plasmodium falciparum* malaria on pregnancy and perinatal outcome in sub-Saharan Africa: I: introduction to placental malaria. Yale J Biol Med 2007; 80(2): 39-50.
[PMID: 18160989]

[33] Błaszkowska J, Góralska K. Parasites and fungi as a threat for prenatal and postnatal human development. Ann Parasitol 2014; 60(4): 225-34.
[PMID: 25706418]

[34] Martins-Melo FR, Lima MdaS, Ramos AN Jr, Alencar CH, Heukelbach J. Prevalence of Chagas disease in pregnant women and congenital transmission of *Trypanosoma cruzi* in Brazil: a systematic review and meta-analysis. Trop Med Int Health 2014; 19(8): 943-57.
[PMID: 24815954]

[35] Carlier Y, Truyens C, Deloron P, Peyron F. Congenital parasitic infections: a review. Acta Trop 2012; 121(2): 55-70.
[PMID: 22085916]

[36] Schwandt A, Williams C, Beigi RH. Perinatal transmission of *Trichomonas vaginalis*: a case report. J Reprod Med 2008; 53(1): 59-61.
[PMID: 18251366]

[37] Wendel S. Transfusion transmitted Chagas disease: is it really under control? Acta Trop 2010; 115(1-2): 28-34.
[PMID: 20044970]

[38] Schmunis GA. Epidemiology of Chagas disease in non-endemic countries: the role of international migration. Mem Ins Oswaldo Cruz. Rio de 2007; 102 (Suppl. I): 75-85.

[39] Brouwer EE, van Hellemond JJ, van Genderen PJ, *et al.* A case report of transfusion-transmitted *Plasmodium malariae* from an asymptomatic non-immune traveller. Malar J 2013; 12: 439.
[PMID: 24304475]

[40] Schneider WH. History of blood transfusion in sub-saharan Africa. Transfus Med Rev 2013; 27(1): 21-8.
[PMID: 22981696]

[41] Austin N, Adikaibe E, Ethelbert O, Chioma U, Ekene N. Prevalence and Severity of Malaria Parasitemia among Children Requiring Emergency Blood Transfusion in a Tertiary Hospital in Imo State, Nigeria. Ann Med Health Sci Res 2014; 4(4): 619-23.
[PMID: 25221716]

[42] Lund TC, Hume H, Allain JP, McCullough J, Dzik W. The blood supply in Sub-Saharan Africa: needs, challenges, and solutions. Transfus Apheresis Sci 2013; 49(3): 416-21.
[PMID: 23871466]

[43] Garraud O, Relave J, Flori P, Perraut R. [Post-transfusion malaria: is the risk irreconciliable with biological silence?]. Transfus Clin Biol 2004; 11(2): 87-94.
[PMID: 15120105]

[44] Contreras CE, Pance A, Marcano N, González N, Bianco N. Detection of specific antibodies to *Plasmodium falciparum* in blood bank donors from malaria-endemic and non-endemic areas of Venezuela. Am J Trop Med Hyg 1999; 60(6): 948-53.
[PMID: 10403326]

[45] Fukutani KF, Figueiredo V, Celes FS, *et al.* Serological survey of *Leishmania* infection in blood donors in Salvador, Northeastern Brazil. BMC Infect Dis 2014; 14: 422.
[PMID: 25073468]

[46] Scarlata F, Vitale F, Saporito L, *et al.* Asymptomatic Leishmania infantum/chagasi infection in blood donors of western Sicily. Trans R Soc Trop Med Hyg 2008; 102(4): 394-6.
[PMID: 18321542]

[47] Ates SC, Bagirova M, Allahverdiyev AM, *et al.* Detection of antileishmanial antibodies in blood sampled from blood bank donors in Istanbul. Future Microbiol 2012; 7(6): 773-9.
[PMID: 22702529]

[48] Riera C, Fisa R, Udina M, Gállego M, Portus M. Detection of *Leishmania infantum* cryptic infection in asymptomatic blood donors living in an endemic area (Eivissa, Balearic Islands, Spain) by different diagnostic methods. Trans R Soc Trop Med Hyg 2004; 98(2): 102-10.
[PMID: 14964810]

[49] Walle F, Kebede N, Tsegaye A, Kassa T. Seroprevalence and risk factors for Toxoplasmosis in HIV infected and non-infected individuals in Bahir Dar, Northwest Ethiopia. Parasit Vectors 2013; 6(1): 15.
[PMID: 23324409]

[50] Shaddel M, Mirzaii Dizgah I, Sharif F. The prevalence of toxoplasmosis in Imam Reza Hospital blood bank samples, Tehran, Iran. Transfus Apheresis Sci 2014; 51(2): 181-3.
[PMID: 25219635]

[51] Cura CI, Lattes R, Nagel C, *et al.* Early molecular diagnosis of acute Chagas disease after transplantation with organs from *Trypanosoma cruzi*-infected donors. Am J Transplant 2013; 13(12): 3253-61.
[PMID: 24266974]

[52] Sever MS, Kazancioğlu R, Yildiz A, *et al.* Outcome of living unrelated (commercial) renal transplantation. Kidney Int 2001; 60(4): 1477-83.
[PMID: 11576362]

[53] Menichetti F, Bindi ML, Tascini C, *et al.* Fever, mental impairment, acute anemia, and renal failure in patient undergoing orthotopic liver transplantation: posttransplantation malaria. Liver Transpl 2006; 12(4): 674-6.
[PMID: 16555320]

[54] Fischer L, Sterneck M, Claus M, *et al.* Transmission of malaria tertiana by multi-organ donation. Clin Transplant 1999; 13(6): 491-5.
[PMID: 10617239]

[55] Assi MA, Rosenblatt JE, Marshall WF. Donor-transmitted toxoplasmosis in liver transplant recipients: a case report and literature review. Transpl Infect Dis 2007; 9(2): 132-6.
[PMID: 17461999]

[56] Gharavi MJ, Jalali S, Khademvatan S, Heydari S. Detection of IgM and IgG anti-*Toxoplasma* antibodies in renal transplant recipients using ELFA, ELISA and ISAGA methods: comparison of pre- and post-transplantation status. Ann Trop Med Parasitol 2011; 105(5): 367-71.
[PMID: 21929878]

[57] Castagnini M, Bernazzali S, Ginanneschi C, *et al.* Fatal disseminated toxoplasmosis in a cardiac transplantation with seropositive match for *Toxoplasma*: should prophylaxis be extended? Transpl Immunol 2007; 18(2): 193-7.
[PMID: 18005867]

[58] Strabelli TMV, Siciliano RF, Campos SV, *et al. Toxoplasma gondii* Myocarditis after adult heart transplantation: successful prophylaxis with pyrimethamine. J Trop Med 2012; 2012: 853562.

[59] Antinori S, Cascio A, Parravicini C, Bianchi R, Corbellino M. Leishmaniasis among organ transplant recipients. Lancet Infect Dis 2008; 8(3): 191-9.
[PMID: 18291340]

[60] Basset D, Faraut F, Marty P, *et al.* Visceral leishmaniasis in organ transplant recipients: 11 new cases and a review of the literature. Microbes Infect 2005; 7(13): 1370-5.
[PMID: 16046170]

[61] Simon I, Wissing KM, Del Marmol V, *et al.* Recurrent leishmaniasis in kidney transplant recipients: report of 2 cases and systematic review of the literature. Transpl Infect Dis 2011; 13(4): 397-406.
[PMID: 21281418]

[62] Roustan G, Jiménez JA, Gutiérrez-Solar B, Gallego JL, Alvar J, Patrón M. Post-kala-azar dermal leishmaniasis with mucosal involvement in a kidney transplant recipient: treatment with liposomal amphotericin B. Br J Dermatol 1998; 138(3): 526-8.
[PMID: 9580814]

[63] Singh S. Changing trends in the epidemiology, clinical presentation, and diagnosis of Leishmania-HIV co-infection in India. Int J Infect Dis 2014; 29: 103-12.
[PMID: 25449244]

[64] van Griensven J, Carrillo E, López-Vélez R, Lynen L, Moreno J. Leishmaniasis in immunosuppressed individuals. Clin Microbiol Infect 2014; 20(4): 286-99.
[PMID: 24450618]

[65] Eza DE, Lucas SB. Fulminant toxoplasmosis causing fatal pneumonitis and myocarditis. HIV Med 2006; 7(6): 415-20.
[PMID: 16903988]

[66] Coelho L, Cardoso SW, Amancio RT, *et al.* Trends in AIDS-defining opportunistic illnesses incidence over 25 years in Rio de Janeiro, Brazil. PLoS One 2014; 9(6): e98666.
[PMID: 24901419]

[67] Laufer MK, van Oosterhout JJ, Thesing PC, *et al.* Impact of HIV-associated immunosuppression on malaria infection and disease in Malawi. J Infect Dis 2006; 193(6): 872-8.

[PMID: 16479522]

[68] Bharti AR, Saravanan S, Madhavan V, *et al.* Correlates of HIV and malaria co-infection in Southern India. Malar J 2012; 11: 306.
[PMID: 22943054]

[69] Ferreira MS, Nishioka SdeA, Silvestre MT, Borges AS, Nunes-Araújo FR, Rocha A. Reactivation of Chagas' disease in patients with AIDS: report of three new cases and review of the literature. Clin Infect Dis 1997; 25(6): 1397-400.
[PMID: 9431385]

[70] Kissinger P, Adamski A. Trichomoniasis and HIV interactions: a review. Sex Transm Infect 2013; 89(6): 426-33.
[PMID: 23605851]

[71] Huang Z, Tatem AJ. Global malaria connectivity through air travel. Malar J 2013; 12: 269.
[PMID: 23914776]

[72] O'Brien SF, Delage G, Seed CR, *et al.* The epidemiology of imported malaria and transfusion policy in 5 nonendemic countries. Transfus Med Rev 2015; 29(3): 162-71.
[PMID: 25933591]

[73] Castellanos ME, Díaz S, Parsons E, *et al.* First imported *Plasmodium ovale* malaria in Central America: case report of a Guatemalan soldier and a call to improve its accurate diagnosis. Mil Med Res 2015; 2: 3.
[PMID: 25722882]

[74] Mouchet J. Airport malaria : a rare disease still poorly understood. Euro Surveill 2000; 5(7): 75-6.
[PMID: 12631851]

[75] Lusina D, Legros F, Esteve V, Klerlein M, Giacomini T. Airport malaria : four new cases in suburban Paris during summer 1999. Euro Surveill 2000; 5(7): 76-80.
[PMID: 12631852]

[76] Siala E, Gamara D, Kallel K, *et al.* Airport malaria: report of four cases in Tunisia. Malar J 2015; 14: 42.
[PMID: 25626591]

[77] Pomares-Estran C, Delaunay P, Mottard A, *et al.* Atypical aetiology of a conjugal fever: autochthonous airport malaria between Paris and French Riviera: a case report. Malar J 2009; 8: 202.
[PMID: 19698152]

[78] Thang HD, Elsas RM, Veenstra J. Airport malaria: report of a case and a brief review of the literatura. J Med 2002; 60: 41-3.

[79] Whitfield D, Curtis CF, White GB, Targett GA, Warhurst DC, Bradley DJ. Two cases of falciparum malaria acquired in Britain. Br Med J (Clin Res Ed) 1984; 289(6458): 1607-9.
[PMID: 6439340]

[80] Mansueto P, Seidita A, Vitale G, Cascio A. Leishmaniasis in travelers: a literature review. Travel Med Infect Dis 2014; 12(6 Pt A): 563-81.
[PMID: 25287721]

[81] Trück J, Rampton C, Kelly SJ, Kelly D. Visceral leishmaniasis in an infant following a holiday trip to Spain. BMJ 2015. Case Rep 28

[82] Roberts T, Barratt J, Sandaradura I, *et al.* Molecular epidemiology of imported cases of leishmaniasis in Australia from 2008 to 2014. PLoS One 2015; 10(3): e0119212.
[PMID: 25734905]

[83] Bern C, Montgomery SP. Recognizing and reducing the risks of Chagas disease in travelers. J Travel Med 2008; 15(5): 385-6.
[PMID: 19006520]

[84] Flores-Figueroa J, Okhuysen PC, von Sonnenburg F, *et al.* GeoSentinel Surveillance Network. Patterns of illness in travelers visiting Mexico and Central America: the GeoSentinel experience. Clin Infect Dis 2011; 53(6): 523-31.
[PMID: 21832261]

[85] Aroussi A, Vignoles P, Dalmay F, *et al.* Detection of *Toxoplasma gondii* DNA in horse meat from supermarkets in France and performance evaluation of two serological tests. Parasite 2015; 22: 14.
[PMID: 25809058]

[86] Halos L, Thébault A, Aubert D, *et al.* An innovative survey underlining the significant level of contamination by *Toxoplasma gondii* of ovine meat consumed in France. Int J Parasitol 2010; 40(2): 193-200.
[PMID: 19631651]

[87] Dubey JP. Toxoplasmosis in pigs--the last 20 years. Vet Parasitol 2009; 164(2-4): 89-103.
[PMID: 19559531]

[88] Sosa-Estani S, Segura EL. Integrated control of Chagas disease for its elimination as public health problem - A Review. Mem Inst Oswaldo Cruz. Rio de 2015; 110: 289-98.

[89] Waleckx E, Gourbière S, Dumonteil E. Intrusive *versus* domiciliated triatomines and the challenge of adapting vector control practices against Chagas disease. Mem Inst Oswaldo Cruz. Rio de 2015; 110: 324-38.

[90] de Souza W. Chagas' disease: facts and reality. Microbes Infect 2007; 9(4): 544-5.
[PMID: 17336119]

[91] Vassena CV, Picollo MI, Zerba EN. Insecticide resistance in Brazilian *Triatoma infestans* and Venezuelan *Rhodnius prolixus*. Med Vet Entomol 2000; 14(1): 51-5.
[PMID: 10759312]

[92] Campos MC, Leon LL, Taylor MC, Kelly JM. Benznidazole-resistance in *Trypanosoma cruzi*: evidence that distinct mechanisms can act in concert. Mol Biochem Parasitol 2014; 193(1): 17-9.
[PMID: 24462750]

[93] Alarcón de Noya B, Díaz-Bello Z, Colmenares C, *et al.* Update on oral Chagas disease outbreaks in Venezuela: epidemiological, clinical and diagnostic approaches. Mem Inst Oswaldo Cruz. Rio de 2015; 110: 377-86.

[94] Burki T. India's ambition to eliminate visceral leishmaniasis. BMJ 2014; 7: 349-6671.

[95] Dhiman RC, Sen AB. Epidemiology of kala-azar in rural Bihar (India) using village as a component

unit of study. Indian J Med Res 1991; 93: 155-60.
[PMID: 1937592]

[96] Alexander B, Maroli M. Control of phlebotomine sandflies. Med Vet Entomol 2003; 17(1): 1-18.
[PMID: 12680919]

[97] Singh RK, Mittal PK, Dhiman RC. Insecticide susceptibility status of *Phlebotomus argentipes*, a vector of visceral leishmaniasis in different foci in three states of India. J Vector Borne Dis 2012; 49(4): 254-7.
[PMID: 23428526]

[98] Sinha S, Medhi B, Sehgal R. Challenges of drug-resistant malaria. Parasite 2014; 21: 61.
[PMID: 25402734]

[99] Vakis R, Rigolini J, Lucchetti L. Los olvidados: pobreza crónica en América Latina y el Caribe. Washington: Banco Mundial 2015.

[100] Coura JR, Borges-Pereira J. Chagas disease: 100 years after its discovery. A systemic review. Acta Trop 2010; 115(1-2): 5-13.
[PMID: 20382097]

[101] Schmunis GA, Cruz JR. Safety of the blood supply in Latin America. Clin Microbiol Rev 2005; 18(1): 12-29.
[PMID: 15653816]

[102] Strasen J, Williams T, Ertl G, Zoller T, Stich A, Ritter O. Epidemiology of Chagas disease in Europe: many calculations, little knowledge. Clin Res Cardiol 2014; 103(1): 1-10.
[PMID: 23989652]

[103] Hotez PJ, Dumonteil E, Betancourt Cravioto M, *et al.* An unfolding tragedy of Chagas disease in North America. PLoS Negl Trop Dis 2013; 7(10): e2300.
[PMID: 24205411]

[104] Alvar J, Yactayo S, Bern C. Leishmaniasis and poverty. Trends Parasitol 2006; 22(12): 552-7.
[PMID: 17023215]

[105] Sutton M, Sternberg M, Koumans EH, McQuillan G, Berman S, Markowitz L. The prevalence of *Trichomonas vaginalis* infection among reproductive-age women in the United States, 2001-2004. Clin Infect Dis 2007; 45(10): 1319-26.
[PMID: 17968828]

[106] Hotez PJ. Neglected infections of poverty in the United States of America. PLoS Negl Trop Dis 2008; 2(6): e256.
[PMID: 18575621]

[107] Alvarado-Esquivel C, Campillo-Ruiz F, Liesenfeld O. Seroepidemiology of infection with *Toxoplasma gondii* in migrant agricultural workers living in poverty in Durango, Mexico. Parasit Vectors 2013; 6: 113.
[PMID: 23601076]

[108] Diaz-Suárez O, Estevez J. Seroepidemiology of toxoplasmosis in women of childbearing age from a marginal community of Maracaibo, Venezuela. Rev Inst Med Trop Sao Paulo 2009; 51(1): 13-7.
[PMID: 19229385]

[109] Francisco FdeM, de Souza SL, Gennari SM, Pinheiro SR, Muradian V, Soares RM. Seroprevalence of toxoplasmosis in a low-income community in the São Paulo municipality, SP, Brazil. Rev Inst Med Trop Sao Paulo 2006; 48(3): 167-70.
[PMID: 16847507]

CHAPTER 2

Drugs for Parasitic Diseases - Strategies to Solve a Global Problem

A. Valeria Pozzoli and **Miriam A. Martins Alho***

LabMOr-INTECIN, Departamento de Química de la Facultad de Ingeniería de la Universidad de Buenos Aires, Ciudad Autónoma de Buenos Aires, Argentina

Abstract: For many years, one of the driving forces for the development of drugs has been, and still is, the pharmaceutical industry, but the need for therapeutic agents regarding unprofitable diseases makes necessary a change in this situation. Parasitic diseases are a good example since the quantity and safety of many drugs currently in use are inadequate, and the development of new agents is insufficient. In the paper herein, we discuss the main methodologies used for the development and discovery of antiparasitics, the new trends and prospects, as well as the first results achieved by supranational programs and consortia created for such purposes.

Keywords: New approaches, New drugs, Parasitic diseases.

INTRODUCTION

Parasitic diseases are a major socioeconomic challenge either affecting humans or animals. They do not only pose a huge health risk, but also limit the proper development of the affected communities, which, in some cases, represent a large part of the population. Apart from the obvious health risks, these infections have a direct impact on the economic development of the population. Humans affected by certain chronic parasitoses typically develop comorbidities which, either directly or indirectly, affect their quality of life, reduce their productive capacity and limit their potential for economic progress. Moreover, parasitic diseases also affect animals that are in direct or indirect contact with humans. The existence

* **Corresponding author Miriam A. Martins Alho:** LabMOr-INTECIN, Facultad de Ingeniería, Paseo Colón 850, 5.° Piso, CABA, Argentina; Tel/Fax: 54 11 4343 0893 E-mail: miriam.alho@gmail.com

Norma Rivera (Ed.)

of infected animals, which are, in some cases, a reservoir allowing these diseases to spread, is also a severe economic damage and results in the loss of animals because they are sacrificed in order to prevent the disease from spreading. Perhaps this is the reason why the parasitic diseases of animals have received comparatively more attention than those of humans from pharmaceutical companies [1].

Part of the lack of interest in human parasitic diseases has been a logical consequence of the roles adopted by different actors in the discovery and development of drugs. Remarkably, the pharmaceutical industry has usually been in charge of said developments, and these companies are profit-driven commercial enterprises. The benefits provided by the commercialization of these drugs do not normally compensate for the large investments needed to develop antiparasitic agents, especially because these diseases are restricted to developing countries with little funding for public health. According to Doctors without borders/Médecins Sans Frontières (MSF), the treatment cost for visceral leishmaniasis is US$450 per patient in their program in India, but this price can climb to US$2,500 per patient, which is too expensive for most government Ministries of Health [2]. This is one of the reasons why parasitic diseases have historically been considered "orphan diseases". The scarce attention received depends exclusively on the academy and/or special programs of either international organizations or nonprofit foundations. Even the resources provided by foundations and nonprofit entities are modest compared to those allocated to the study of other diseases, such as HIV. These huge differences derive from the lack of visibility of parasitic diseases, even when they incapacitate millions of people annually. The World Health Organization (WHO) includes some parasitoses, such as Chagas disease, human African trypanosomiasis (HAT, or sleeping sickness) and leishmaniasis, within the Neglected Tropical Diseases (NTDs). According to the WHO, NTDs do not only affect millions of people across 149 countries, deriving in high costs for developing economies, but also have a high mortality rate if they are not treated properly [2].

In a publication of 2013, Jaggi reported that in the last 20 years the Food and Drug Administration (FDA) has approved 1,200 new drugs and only 3 of them are antiparasitics. Furthermore, not only are there few new antiparasitic drugs, but, considering the time needed for such drugs to reach the market, there is no prospect either for new alternatives to appear in the near future [3]. This lack of new antiparasitic agents means that drugs developed between 1930 and 1970 are still in use. The constant use of these drugs since then has led to resistance phenomena, thereby reducing their effectiveness. However, the international interest in parasitic diseases is growing because the global landscape of infections is changing. There are two main factors driving this change:

- *The increase in the area of influence of parasitic diseases:* The recrudescence of situations generating social, economic, ethnic, religious and/or political tension turns the migrant issue into a problem difficult to solve. There are thousands of people displaced from their usual areas of residence, leaving behind their past in search of better places to live. In these mass movements, other less obvious "immigrants" come along, which should not be neglected. On the other hand, many people in developed countries travel around the globe, both for professional reasons and out of a desire to visit new places, exposing themselves to health risks which are unusual in their places of residence. In a few words, globalization is also a driving force for the spread of parasitic diseases. The truth is that the emergence of new areas affected by parasites (outside their endemic regions) does not only have an impact on developed countries. In some cases, they are the "exporters" of parasitosis. In Argentina, there have been cases of infections with *Diphyllobothrium latum,* a tapeworm of salmonids found in Canada and Japan, which has apparently been introduced during the planting of trouts. Moreover, in the City of Buenos Aires, an increase of parasitosis has also been verified in recent years, previously rare in said area, along with an increasing incidence of infections with *Taenia saginata* and *Taenia solium*, including the development of cases of neurocysticercosis [4].

While this "importation" of pathologies is often limited to affected individuals, if the parasite finds the appropriate proliferation medium, such as poor hygiene, or the appropriate vectors are present, it can quickly become a mass phenomenon. Regardless of the obvious concern for global health, the increase of people affected by parasites makes this issue more interesting for the pharmaceutical industry. As for the availability of vectors, there is a change that is related to the second factor:

- *Climate change*: The tropicalization of different areas formerly considered as temperate is making the emergence of vectors in unconventional areas possible. Once the vector is installed in the zone, the presence of repositories completes the picture for the emergence of a new region affected by the parasite.

Facing this new situation, the emergence of new antiparasitics can no longer depend exclusively on the interests of the pharmaceutical industry, but the response capacity of academia is not consistent with the urgency of the times. This predicament has resulted in a new paradigm regarding R&D projects: cooperation between the pharmaceutical industry and academic organizations, as well as contributions of private support (foundations, philanthropic entities and individual contributions). On this synergistic interaction is currently based the best hope of finding new tools against parasitic diseases.

THE CHALLENGE OF PARASITIC DISEASES

The fight against parasitic diseases is usually a difficult problem as it presents different aspects. While both defunding (low investment in R&D) and the lack of new therapeutic agents are a serious obstacle, this is only one side of the coin. The lack of preventive measures, including appropriate and consistent health policies, often aggravates the situation. Some of the preventive measures that were successful in the past are related to improving sanitary conditions of the population, access to safe drinking water and containment of transmission vectors. Although these practices are normally limited to urban areas, they drastically reduce the incidence of diseases if prolonged in time on a regular and constant basis. All these measures depend on governmental decisions, and only on rare occasions they are considered thoroughly as state policies, so their continuity over time is often seriously compromised.

Another challenge is related to the characteristics of the parasite itself. Even when counting with adequate resources, the complexity of the life cycle of certain parasites often makes it difficult to locate a suitable therapeutic target. When it is possible to obtain an active compound, it generally acts on one or two stages of the pathogen. As a consequence, prolonged treatments are required in order to cover, with a certain margin, the entire life cycle of the parasite and prevent reinfections. This type of prolonged treatment increases the risk of abandonment on the part of the patient, not only due to the lack of consistency, but also because of its side effects. Benznidazole and nifurtimox, for example, are the only choice available for the treatment of patients with Chagas disease. The use of these drugs usually causes pruritic macular rash, gastrointestinal disorders, such as nausea, vomiting and diarrhea, and also polyneuropathies, dizziness, headache and fever, epigastric pain and disturbances both in the peripheral and central nervous systems, insomnia and polyneuritis, among other side effects [5]. Other antiparasitic drugs are not exempt from side effects, and even teratogenicity [6 - 26], so it is imperative to find effective drugs which do not compromise the patient's general condition. A summary of currently used antiparasitic drugs is showed in Table **1**.

Table 1. Most commonly used drugs, parasitosis in which they are used and their target in the pathogen.

Drug	Parasitosis	Target
Albendazole Mebendazole	Ancylostoma. Ascariasis. Hookworms and Tapeworms. Microsporidiosis. Trichinellosis. Strongyloidiasis.	Inhibitory effect on tubulin polymerization, which results in the loss of cytoplasmic microtubules. Inhibitor of protein tubulin b-2 chain.
Amphotericin	Leishmaniasis.	Interaction with membrane sterols of promastigote cells. It affects the permeability barrier for small metabolites. Interaction with cholesterol of host membranes.
Artesunate	Malaria (*P. falciparum* in chloroquine-resistant areas).	Inhibition of EXP1, a parasitic membrane glutathione *S*-transferase which degrades cytotoxic hematin.
Artemether	Malaria (All *Plasmodium*).	Interaction with ferriprotoporphyrin IX, or ferrous ions, in the acidic parasite food vacuole.
Atovaquone	Malaria (*P.falciparum*, chloroquine-resistant). Pneumocystis.	Cytochrome bc1. Selective interference of mitochondrial redox reactions, like ATP biosynthesis.
Benznidazole	Trypanosomiasis (*T. cruzi*).	It generates free radicals. Covalent binding of the nitro reduction intermediaries with components of the parasite, like DNA, lipids and proteins.
Chloroquine	Malaria (All *Plasmodium*, except for chloroquine-resistant).	It produces an accumulation of free heme, probably by inhibition of heme polymerase activity. The heme-chloroquine complex disrupts membrane function and produces cell lysis.

(Table 1) contd.....

Drug	Parasitosis	Target
Eflornithine	Trypanosomiasis (*T. brucei gambiense*).	It irreversibly inhibits the ornithine decarboxylase which catalyzes the biosynthesis of polyamines.
Iodoquinol	Amebiasis.	Contact amebicide that works in the lumen of the intestine by an unknown mechanism.
Ivermectin	Ascariasis. Scabies. Strongyloidiasis.	It binds selectively to glutamate-gated chloride ion channels in muscle and nerve cells of the microfilaria. It produces hyperpolarization of the cell, leading to paralysis and death of the parasite. Ivermectin is also believed to act as an agonist of GABA, thereby disrupting GABA-mediated central nervous system (CNS) neurosynaptic transmission.
Melarsoprol	Trypanosomiasis (*T. brucei gambiense*).	It reacts with trypanothione, forming a competitive inhibitor of trypanothione reductase.
Metronidazole	Amebiasis. Giardiasis. Trichomoniasis.	It is a prodrug. Anaerobic bacteria reduce metronidazole to its active form intracellularly. This reduced metronidazole then covalently binds to DNA, disrupts its helical structure, inhibiting nucleic acid synthesis and resulting in bacterial cell death.
Nifurtimox	Trypanosomiasis (*T. cruzi*).	The mode of action is not clearly known. It may be related to the generation of reactive oxygen species which damage cellular components, such as DNA, membrane lipids and proteins.
Nitazoxanide	Ascariasis. Cryptosporidiosis. *Fasciola hepatica*. Giardiasis. Tapeworms.	The antiprotozoal activity of nitazoxanide is believed to be the result of the interference with the pyruvate: ferredoxin oxidoreductase (PFOR) enzyme-dependent electron transfer reaction, which is essential to anaerobic energy metabolism.
Pentamidine	Leishmaniasis. Pneumocystis. Trypanosomiasis (*T. brucei gambiense*).	The mode of action of pentamidine is not fully understood. The drug probably interferes with the nuclear metabolism producing inhibition of the synthesis of DNA, RNA, phospholipids and proteins.
Praziquantel	Schistosomiasis. Tapeworms.	The mode of action is not exactly known. The tapeworm loses its ability to resist digestion by the mammalian host. Schistosome calcium ion channels are currently the only known targets of praziquantel.
Pyrimethamine	Toxoplasmosis. Malaria.	It inhibits the dihydrofolate reductase of the parasite.
Quinine	Malaria (*P. vivax*, chloroquine-resistant).	It interferes with the parasite's ability to break down and digest hemoglobin. The parasite starves and/or builds up toxic levels of partially degraded hemoglobin in itself.
Sodium Stibogluconate	Leishmaniasis.	It inhibits DNA topoisomerase I leading to inhibition of both DNA replication and transcription.

(Table 1) contd.....

Drug	Parasitosis	Target
Suramin	Trypanosomiasis (*T. brucei gambiense*).	The mechanism is unknown. The trypanocidal activity may be the result of the inhibition of enzymes involved in the oxidation of NADH, which functions as a co-enzyme in many cellular reactions.

DISCOVERING PARASITIC DRUGS

Drug Design Based on Nature

Leaving aside accidental discoveries, the search to find new drugs can take different paths. One of the most traditional strategies is the isolation and characterization of bioactive agents from natural products. The next step is the optimization of properties in order to obtain synthetic and/or semisynthetic analogs from these natural bioactive agents.

In fact, one of the first antimalarial agents to be used was quinine, which emerged from traditional American medicine. This active principle is present in decoctions of the cinchona tree bark (quina). It was used by the original inhabitants of the Peruvian Andes region to treat fevers, there being news of its use since the 17th century [27]. Another "rediscovered" drug, coming from traditional medicines, is artemisinin or qinghaosu. This drug is a sesquiterpene lactone which was used in traditional Chinese medicine for various purposes about 150 years BC, and it was rediscovered in 1972 as an antimalarial agent [28]. Due to solubility, stability and administration problems regarding artemisinin, artesunate and artemether were subsequently developed (Fig. **1**). During the 80s, it was discovered, by serendipity, that artemether has a broad spectrum of action against various trematodes, such a human schistosomes, *Clonorchis sinensis*, *Fasciola hepatica* and *Opisthorchis viverrini* [29]. Artemisinin has also shown promising effects on visceral leishmaniasis, especially in cases where the usual treatment with antimonials (sodium stibogluconate and glucantime) does not offer good results [30].

Natural products and popular medicines from different regions of the world are still of interest, even in the 21st century. Bahmani *et al.* conducted an analysis concerning different types of herbs used as antiparasitic in some regions of Iran, although neither the determination of active ingredients nor the effectiveness of said herbs has been reported [31, 32]. In 2011, Bolivar *et al.* published a study on the antimicrobial, antiparasitic and anti-inflammatory effects of a plant used in traditional Mexican medicine, the *Galium Mexicanum* [33], and this year, Christensen *et al.* carried out a study on the activity of 21 plants from Ghana, frequently used as a decoction for relieving stomach disorders, such as diarrhea and dysentery. While they did not perform an identification of the active compounds, the anti-blastocystis action was evaluated [34]. In recent literature, other examples of extensive work on the antiparasitic activity of some natural products and their derivatives can be found [35 - 38].

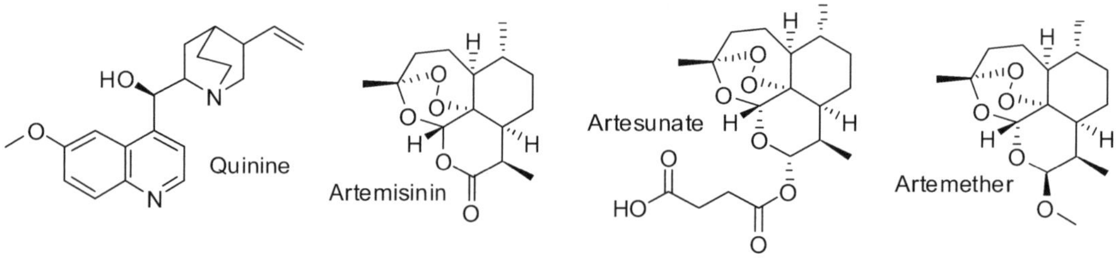

Fig. (1). Chemical structures for quinine, artemisinin and their derivatives.

Developments Based on Structural Similarity

In order to find new therapeutic agents, it is usual to start from the basis that similar structures should have a similar biological behavior. Based on the structure of quinine (and methylene blue), in the early 30s, two new active synthetic drugs were found: chloroquine (a quinoline) and quinacrine (an acridine) [39]. Indeed, chloroquine still remains as the drug of choice, except for the treatment of resistant strains of *Plasmodium falciparum* and *Plasmodium vivax* [40]. A further development (in the 70s) led to mefloquine, which shares a quinoline core with its predecessors. Another parasite which also contains a quinoline in its structure is iodoquinol, developed in the 60s and used for the treatment of infections with Dientamoeba fragilis. Their chlorinated analog, chloroquine, was withdrawn in 1970 due to cases of neurotoxicity being registered in Japan (Fig. **2**) [41].

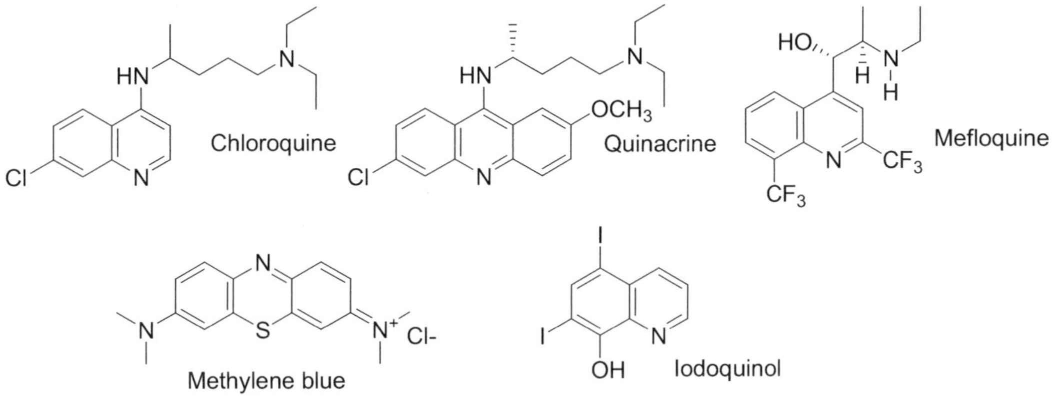

Fig. (2). Chemical structures for methylene blue, quinoline and acridine antiparasitic drugs.

Recently, Pérez-Villanueva *et al.* analyzed the *in vitro* activity of benzimidazole drugs currently used in therapeutics as proton pump inhibitors (PPIs) (omeprazole, lanzoprazole, pantoprazole and rabeprazole). The choice was based on their structural similarity with mebendazole and albendazole, known antiparasitic drugs from the azole family. They found a good activity against *T. vaginalis*, *G. intestinalis* and *E. histolytica*, and in some cases, it even surpassed the activity of metronidazole [42] (Fig. **3**). As it can be seen, structural similarity can still be a useful resource for searching and finding leader compounds, but, perhaps, this last case could be better classified as drug redirecting.

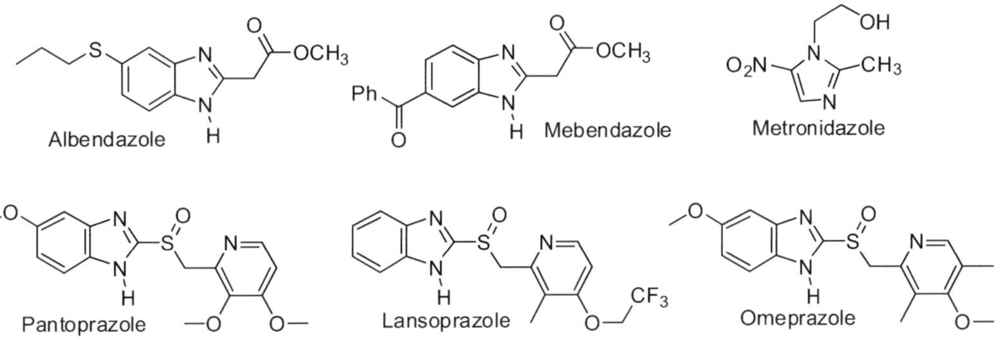

Fig. (3). Chemical structures for quinine, antiparasitics and some proton pump inhibitors.

Redirecting Drugs

Another approach for the discovery of new antiparasitic agents is the redirection of drugs. This strategy uses drugs approved for other therapeutic targets or molecules from another pharmaceutical development and tests their effects on various parasites. A successful example of the redirection of drugs is the use of eflornithine to treat HAT. The usual treatment was based on the same drugs for forty years (suramin, melarsoprol and pentamidine) until the FDA, in the 90s, approved the use of eflornithine, a drug originally developed in the 70s for cancer treatment and used for the treatment of hirsutism. On the other hand, some antibiotics like paromomycin, azithromycin, spiramycin and amphotericin B are used for the treatment of several parasitoses [40] (Fig. **4**). The last three are glycosylated macrocyclic lactones and have a structural similarity with the antiparasitic drug ivermectin.

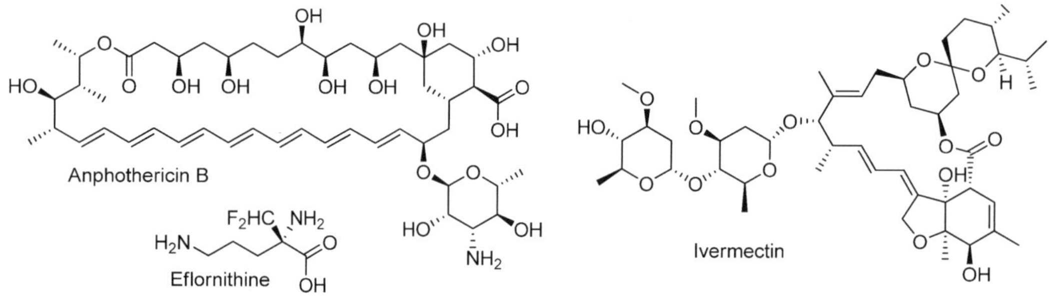

Fig. (4). Chemical structures for eflornithine, amphotericin B and ivermectin.

Some years ago, a number of selected bisphosphonates, including the FDA-approved drugs for osteoporosis treatment, pamidronate and alendronate, were found to be potent inhibitors of *Trypanosoma cruzi*, *in vitro* and *in vivo*, with no toxicity to the host cells [43]. Another common practice in drug research is to use a therapeutic target which has been studied for oncology applications and evaluate it for other pharmacological applications. The Hsp90 is a cytosolic molecular chaperone, essential for protein homeostasis and activation of many signaling molecules studied in other diseases. Inhibitors of Hsp90 yielded interesting results when they were tested against *Trypanosoma brucei rhodesiense* and *Plasmodium falciparum* [44].

The Rational Design

In the early 90s, the application of combinatorial chemistry & high-throughput screening became popular because it allowed for the synthesis and evaluation of a large number of compounds in a short time. Many hopes were put in this methodology because it made it possible to develop new drugs much faster than expected when applying the traditional way. While this type of approach has reported great progress in obtaining peptides and nucleotides using techniques of solid phase synthesis, some people believe that, in the field of small molecules, it has not yet fulfilled the expectations placed on it [45 - 47].

However, taking into account that the different evaluation stages for new drugs are very expensive procedures, the trend of high-throughput screening remains valid. This methodology is used to build rationally designed libraries from the identification of therapeutic targets and the study of the structure-activity relationships (SAR). A rational approach for the synthesis of antiparasitics is to identify targets in the parasite (target-based screening) and design inhibitors of the expression of different proteins or blockers of certain metabolic steps. However, both the quantity and performance of antiparasitics resulting so far from this method have been poor since the inhibition of protein synthesis does not necessarily interfere with the parasite biology [48]. In the case of trypanosomatids for example, it has been determined that there is a specific requirement for endogenous sterols, and the parasite is unable to use the sterols of the mammalian host. The inhibitors of ergosterol biosynthesis possess potent *in vitro* activity and special pharmacokinetic properties in mammals, so they could lead to the cure in animal models of both acute and chronic Chagas disease [49]. Squalene synthase is an enzyme involved in the biosynthesis of sterols inhibited by Phenoxy-phenoxyethyl thiocyanate. Based on this information, Elicio *et al.* used Phenoxyphenoxyethyl thiocyanate as the leading drug in order to design and synthesize a new series of inhibitors for the enzyme using SAR [50]. According to K. R. Matthews, a representative milestone for the understanding of this infection is the development of molecular parasitology. He considers that important discoveries are being made from molecular parasitology and their relative weight on the emergence of new therapies is only now beginning to have an impact [51].

The literature accounts for numerous efforts to understand the different mechanisms involved in certain antiparasitic activities, many of them using computer-assisted methods. Recently, Stolfa *et al.* studied the molecular basis for the inhibition of histone deacetylase 8 in *Schistosoma mansoni*, and Chaal *et al.* conducted a study regarding histone deacetylase inhibitors in *Plasmodium falciparum* [52, 53]. In addition, Shibi and co-workers published a computational study on a big series of aminoquinoline derivatives in order to understand the antimalarial properties using techniques of molecular modeling and docking [54]. According to the authors, this study provides useful guidelines for developing 7-substituted-4-aminoquinoline derivatives as potent antimalarials.

The use of computer-assisted molecular design is an intelligent alternative in all the stages of drug discovery. For Scalese *et al.*, the QSAR study led to a design guide for the development of new active compounds, with improved biological profiles. In their work, they carried out computational modeling in order to compare the ability of each of six series of complexes with different co-ligands to intercalate DNA, using molecular docking [55]. The computational tools for drug design are a powerful source of new ideas, which facilitate and direct the experimental results. This topic is developed elsewhere in this book.

PERSPECTIVES

As it was mentioned before, a different methodology has emerged over the last few years as a new paradigm for the search and development of new drugs for Neglected Diseases. Several organizations have taken up the challenge of developing new antiparasitic agents, acting as linkers between all the stakeholders involved in the process. This approach optimizes the exchange of information, the allocation of resources, the coordination of the activity tests and, eventually, the delivery to the public. Some entities, such as the Drugs for Neglected Diseases Initiative and the Consortium for Parasitic Drug Development are part of more than one single program. As a result, there is a mutual collaboration between different initiatives in order to exchange information on drug research and discovery projects for the purpose of avoiding redundancy and sharing their knowledge. The Drugs for Neglected Diseases Initiative (DNDi, www.dndi.org) has defined itself as a collaborative, patient's needs-driven, and not-for-profit drug

R&D organization that is developing new treatments for Neglected Diseases. As it declares in its own homepage, it launched six new treatments between 2006 and 2010, two for malaria, one for HAT, two for visceral leishmaniasis and an adaptation of Chagas treatment for children. Besides, it has announced thirteen candidates for new drugs in clinical stage.

While the DNDi works on a broader spectrum of parasitosis, the Consortium for Parasitic Drug Development (CPDD, www.thecpdd.org), which was set up in 2000, is devoted to the discovery and development of new drugs for HAT and visceral leishmaniasis. The CPDD starts from lead optimization through clinical trials and registration. This organization is made up by professionals from academic and nonprofit private institutions. Another two of these organizations, focused on one or a few diseases, are Medicines for Malaria Venture (MMV, www.mmv.org) and the NGBS Consortium. MMV has been working since 1999 and it has defined itself as a not-for-profit public-private partnership, with more than 375 partners in the last 10 years, in over 50 countries from the public sector, from the private sector, from NGOs and nonprofit organizations, as well as from clinical centers. On the other hand, The NGBS Consortium is a malaria drug discovery program resulting from the collaboration between Novartis Institute for Tropical Diseases (NITD), the Genomics Institute of the Novartis Research Foundation (GNF), the Biomedical Primate Research Centre (BPRC) and the Swiss Tropical and Public Health Institute (Swiss TPH).

As it can be inferred from the information above, the parasitosis which is in the spotlight is malaria and there are many reasons for that. One of them is the large number of immigrants from affected areas who constantly arrive in Europe, thereby increasing not only health risks, but also public concern. Moreover, despite having more therapeutic agents than other parasitoses, the tendency of *P. falciparum* to become drug resistant derives in the number of new candidates never being enough. Flanery *et al.* published in 2013 that there were eight drugs in preclinical stage and other nine in Phase I, II or III [56]. These new drugs come from a great variety of chemical families (triazolopyrimidines, pyrazoles, aminopyridines, imidazolopiperidines, *etc.*) and, remarkably, among Phase III, there are two extracts of natural products. One is extracted from *Argemone mexicana* (successfully used as first line of defense against malaria in Mali, with similar results to artesunate-amodiaquine treatment) [57, 58], and the other comes from *Nauclea pobeguinii*, less tolerable than artesunate-amodiaquine, but with less collateral effects [59].

Two families with promising activity for the treatment of malaria are spiroindolones and imidazole piperazines. These findings are the result of the research carried out by the NGBS Consortium, which worked with two different strategies. Spiroindolones were found by *in vitro* screening of a library of more than 12,000 natural and synthetic compounds with structural features of natural products. Based on the reactivity of each compound, the spiroindolone base structure was selected and optimized, and NITD609 was subsequently found [60, 61]. For the imidazolopiperazine family, they identified possible targets and conducted a high-throughput screening so as to identify new chemotypes, which were then refined using SAR techniques [62]. The compounds resulting from these investigations (NITD609 and GNF156, Fig. **5**) are now under evaluation.

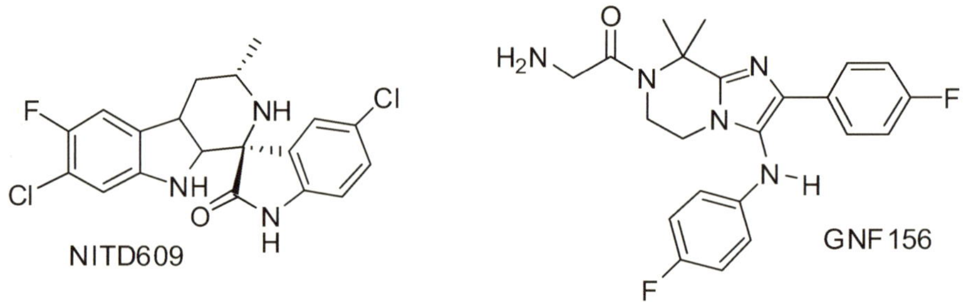

Fig. (5). Chemical structures for NITD609 and GNF156.

When analyzing the different drugs introduced for the treatment of malaria since 1970, we can see that artemisinin was the last one to develop resistance [48]. Artemisinin, a sesquiterpene lactone with an endoperoxide bridge, has an extremely short half-life and, consequently, two daily administrations are necessary. Looking for a better pharmacokinetics, the University of Nebraska Medical Center, the Swiss TPH and the Centre for Drug Candidate Optimization (Melbourne) synthesized a great number of adamantane ozonides, which had good activity and selectivity *in vitro*. As a result of these investigations, they obtained OZ277, known as arterolane, and it was registered in India for combinatorial therapy for malaria. Another discovery resulting from this program is OZ439 (Fig. **6**). According to MMV, this drug is a great candidate for a single-dose treatment for malaria because it exhibits a prolonged blood concentration in volunteer patients, a good tolerance to 1,600 mg doses and a rapid reduction in parasitemia was verified both for *P. falciparum* and *P. vivax* [63].

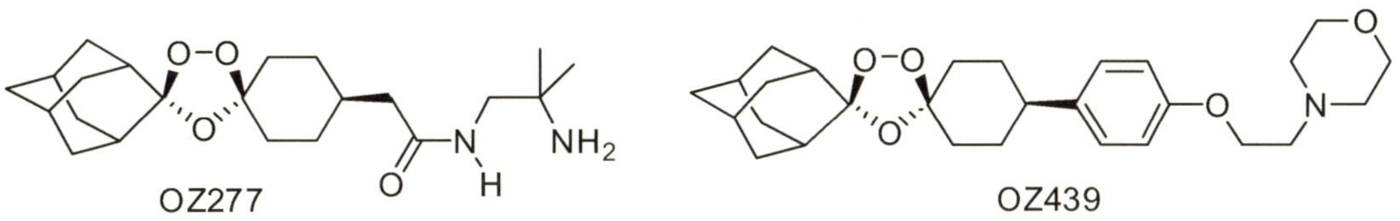

Fig. (6). Chemical structures for OZ277 and OZ439.

Last year, GlaxoSmithKline and MMV announced the start of a Phase III global program to evaluate the efficacy and safety of tafenoquine, a drug from the quinoline family, which is being developed for the treatment and relapse prevention (radical cure) of *P. vivax*. This compound is an analog of primaquine, but with a pharmacokinetic profile that allows for a single-dose therapy regarding relapse prevention *versus* the 14-day regimen required with primaquine [48].

Other products which are being tested as antimalarials are DSM265 (MMV, Phase II, https://clinicaltrials.gov/ct2/show/NCT02123290) and ELQ-300, a potent and selective inhibitor not only of the parasite cytochrome bc1 complex at blood stages of the parasite, but also of the forms that are crucial for disease transmission (Fig. **7**). The first results are expected for 2016 [64].

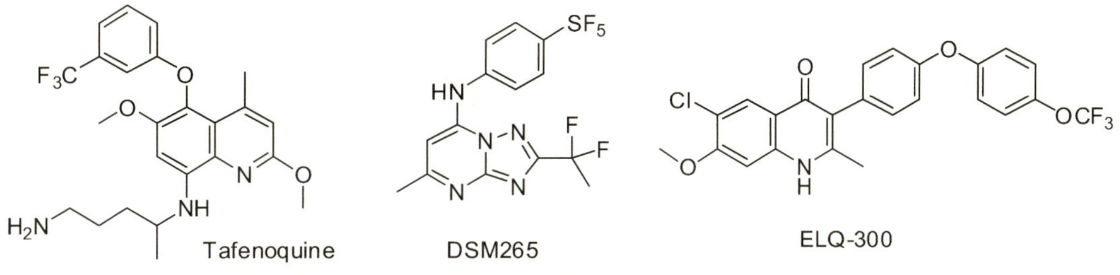

Fig. (7). Chemical structures for tafenoquine, DSM265 and ELQ-300.

In the field of HAT treatment, the drug of choice is still pentamidine, a drug introduced in 1941 [65]. Based on this, the CPDD has screened over 2,000 new diamidines against *T. brucei,* and an initial lead (DB75) was refined into the prodrug DB289 (pafuramidine) (Fig. **8**), efficient against the parasite and having characteristics of blood-brain barrier penetration. This was the first trypanocide to reach clinical tests as an oral drug [66]. The development of DB289 was discontinued in 2008, due to adverse effects, such as liver toxicity and kidney insufficiency in Phase I patients, but the reasons for this behavior are still under investigation.

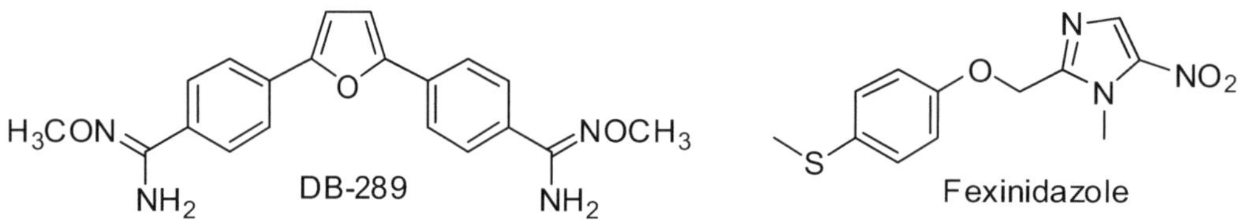

Fig. (8). Chemical structures for prodrug DB-289 and fexinidazole.

Better luck had the efforts of the DNDi in the extensive search for compounds within the nitroimidazole project initiated in 2005. As nifurtimox, combined with eflornithine, is used for a later stage of HAT, the DNDi started screening a large number of nitroimidazole compounds and, as a consequence, it found fexinidazole (Fig. **8**). This drug is produced by Hoechst as an antimicrobial agent, which results to be active against *T. brucei.* According to recent reports, fexinidazole is well tolerated in doses up to 1,800 mg a day for a period of four days, followed by a dose of 1,200 mg for six days. It is expected that the systemic concentration obtained can be clinically effective and administered safely against both stages of HAT [67].

A new kind of organic structure is rising on the horizon of antiparasitic agents: the oxaboroles. These compounds are a new class of antimicrobials developed by Anacor Pharmaceuticals. A review of the oxaboroles library allowed for the finding of a leader compound, which was optimized and SCYX-7158 was obtained as a result (Fig. **9**). This drug has good oral bioavailability as well as good hematoencephalic permeability. Its efficacy and pharmacokinetic properties make it a promising candidate for the treatment of stage II of HAT [68]. As to reports of the DNDi, studies on volunteers started in 2013, but they were suspended because the half-life times in human plasma were higher than expected. A restart was scheduled for the same year but, until now, there have not been new published results.

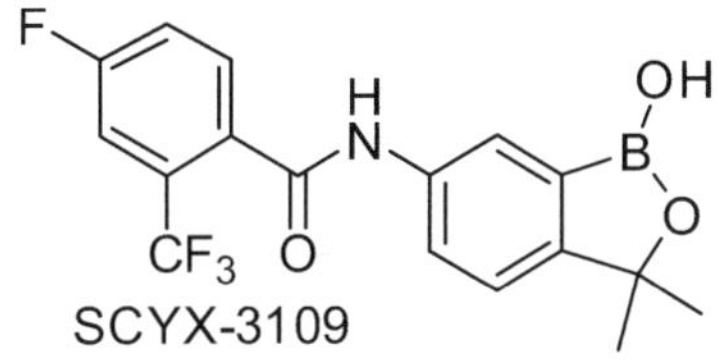

Fig. (9). Chemical structures for oxaborole SCYX-3109.

As it can be seen from the information above, some new alternatives are emerging for malaria, even for HAT. Other parasitic diseases are not so lucky, though, and only a few initiatives are devoted to them. They are forgotten among the neglected. Leishmaniasis is treated with pentavalent antimonial compounds, such as sodium stibogluconate, a drug from the 40s, alone or in combination with paromomycin. Some azoles (ketoconazole, itraconazole and fluconazole) are used as drugs for leishmania with different results [69].

In 1997, amphotericin B was approved for visceral leishmaniasis treatment, but there was no news until 2014, when the FDA approved the oral agent miltefosine for both cutaneous and visceral leishmaniasis. Miltefosine was included in the WHO essential medicines list as an antileishmaniasis medicine in March 2011 [70]. Schistosomiasis is effectively treated with praziquantel (Fig. **10**), a drug available since the mid-70s, but fearing the emergence of resistant strains, other alternatives are being evaluated [71].

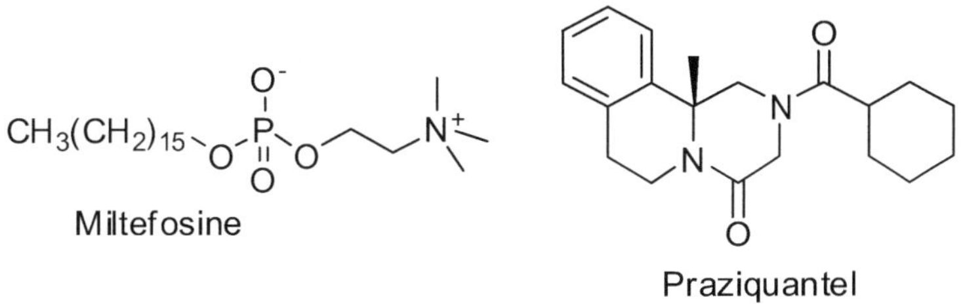

Fig. (10). Chemical structures for miltefosine and praziquantel.

Currently, Chagas is being treated exclusively with benznidazole and nifurtimox. This disease has, by far, the most uncertain prospects for the emergence of new drugs. The preferred therapeutic goal is still the design of inhibitors of ergosterol synthesis, but no promising results have been achieved yet [72, 73]. The DNDi and Eisai Co. Ltd. (a Japanese pharmaceutical company) started to collaborate in 2009 so as to develop a new drug for Chagas disease. E1224 (Fig. **11**) emerged from this interaction, and the Phase II study started in July 2011 in Bolivia. This compound demonstrated a good activity against *T. cruzi*, but it did not offer protection as a single medication and showed some safety issues at high doses, so it is under evaluation in combinatorial treatment for Chagas disease [74].

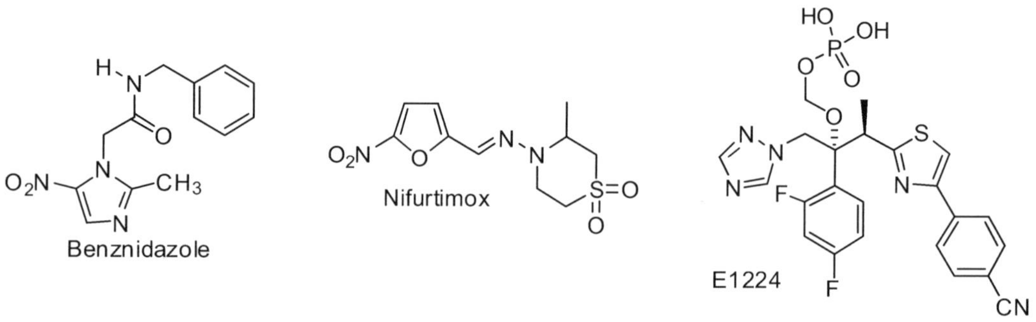

Fig. (11). Chemical structures for benznidazole, nifurtimox and E1224.

CONCLUDING REMARKS

Parasitic diseases have affected millions of people, but, for many years, they have been invisible. Their suffering has been ignored by many, including pharmaceutical companies, governments, researchers and ordinary people. Now, when the problem is about to become a global issue, it is the right time to join efforts across the world using all known strategies and resources. Some people have already begun and, perhaps, the best opportunity for us to solve this problem is to commit ourselves to its resolution, each one making use of its own abilities.

CONFLICT OF INTEREST

The authors confirm that they have no conflict of interest to declare for this publication.

ACKNOWLEDGEMENTS

The authors wish to thank Prof. Dr. Gabriela Razzite for sharing her experiences with us. I would like to thank Prof. Dr. Vicente Arán for making me feel part of his team (MAMA).

GLOSSARY

BC = Before Christ.

CPDD = The Consortium for Parasitic Drug Development.

DNDi = The Drugs for Neglected Diseases Initiative.

FDA = Food and Drug Administration.

HAT = Human African Trypanosomiasis.

HIV = Human immunodeficiency virus.

MMV = Medicines for Malaria Venture.

MSF = Doctors without borders/Médecins Sans Frontières.

NGBS = A public-private partnership of the Novartis Institute for Tropical Diseases, Genomic Institute of the Novartis Research Foundation, Biomedical Primate Research Center and Swiss Tropical and Public Health Institute.

NGOs = Non-Governmental Organizations.

NTDs = Neglected Tropical Diseases.

PPIs = Proton Pump Inhibitors.

QSAR = Quantitative structure-activity relationship.

R&D = Research and Development.

SAR = Structure-Activity Relationships.

WHO = The World Health Organ.

REFERENCES

[1] Geary TG, Thompson DP. Development of antiparasitic drugs in the 21st century. Vet Parasitol 2003; 115(2): 167-84.
[http://dx.doi.org/10.1016/S0304-4017(03)00205-X] [PMID: 12878421]

[2] >Médecins Sans Frontières/Doctors without borders [http://www.msf.org/] 2003. Retrieved from: http://www.doctorswithoutborders.org/sites/usa/files/MSF-NTD-Briefing-Paper.pdf .

[3] Jaggi N. Newer antiparasitic agents. J Patient Saf Infect Control 2013; 1: 27-8.
[http://dx.doi.org/10.1016/S2214-207X(13)11010-6]

[4] Personal communication with Dr. Gabriela Razzite, Head of the Parasitology Unit. J M Ramos Mejía Hospital, CABA, Argentina

[5] Storino R. Enfermedad de Chagas 2005. retrieved from: http://chagasenelsxxi.org.ar/wp-content/uploads/Cardiología-Enfermedad-de-Chagas.pdf.

[6] Iatropoulos MJ, Wang CX, von Keutz E, Williams GM. Assessment of chronic toxicity and carcinogenicity in an accelerated cancer bioassay in rats of Nifurtimox, an anti-trypanosomiasis drug. Exp Toxicol Pathol 2006; 57(5-6): 397-404.
[http://dx.doi.org/10.1016/j.etp.2006.01.005] [PMID: 16616835]

[7] Kijima A, Ishii Y, Takasu S, *et al.* Chemical structure-related mechanisms underlying *in vivo* genotoxicity induced by nitrofurantoin and its constituent moieties in gpt delta rats. Toxicology 2015; 331: 125-35.
[http://dx.doi.org/10.1016/j.tox.2015.03.003] [PMID: 25772432]

[8] Rajasekaran R, Chen YP. Potential therapeutic targets and the role of technology in developing novel antileishmanial drugs 2015. Drug Discov Today 2015; 20(8): 958-68
[http://dx.doi.org/10.1016/j.drudis.2015.04.006]

[9] Rodriguez-Caruncho C, Bielsa Marsol I. Antimalarials in dermatology: mechanism of action, indications, and side effects. Actas Dermosifiliogr 2014; 105(3): 243-52.
[http://dx.doi.org/10.1016/j.adengl.2012.10.021] [PMID: 24656224]

[10] Rosenblatt JE, Edson RS. Symposium on antimicrobial agents. Metronidazole. Mayo Clin Proc 1987; 62(11): 1013-7.
[http://dx.doi.org/10.1016/S0025-6196(12)65074-5] [PMID: 3312851]

[11] Koch-Weser J, Goldman P. Drug therapy: metronidazole. N Engl J Med 1980; 303(21): 1212-8.
[http://dx.doi.org/10.1056/NEJM198011203032106] [PMID: 6999352]

[12] Stahlberg D, Bárány F, Einarsson K, Ursing B, Elmqvist D, Persson A. Neurophysiologic studies of patients with Crohn's disease on long-term treatment with metronidazole. Scand J Gastroenterol 1991; 26(2): 219-24.
[http://dx.doi.org/10.3109/00365529109025034] [PMID: 1849313]

[13] Wienbren M, Perinpanayagam RM, Camba L, Lee CA. Convulsions and encephalopathy in a patient with leukemia after treatment with metronidazole. J Clin Pathol 1985; 38(9): 1076.
[http://dx.doi.org/10.1136/jcp.38.9.1076-b] [PMID: 3862678]

[14] Learned-Coughlin S. Peripheral neuropathy induced by metronidazole. Ann Pharmacother 1994; 28(4): 536.
[PMID: 8038481]

[15] Lawford R, Sorrell TC. Amebic abscess of the spleen complicated by metronidazole-induced neurotoxicity: case report. Clin Infect Dis 1994; 19(2): 346-8.
[http://dx.doi.org/10.1093/clinids/19.2.346] [PMID: 7986915]

[16] Boyce EG, Cookson ET, Bond WS. Persistent metronidazole-induced peripheral neuropathy. DICP 1990; 24(1): 19-21.
[PMID: 2154078]

[17] Schentag JJ, Ziemniak JA, Greco JM, Rainstein M, Buckley RJ. Mental confusion in a patient treated with metronidazole--a concentration-related effect? Pharmacotherapy 1982; 2(6): 384-7.
[http://dx.doi.org/10.1002/j.1875-9114.1982.tb03216.x] [PMID: 7167392]

[18] Beloosesky Y, Grosman B, Marmelstein V, Grinblat J. Convulsions induced by metronidazole treatment for *Clostridium difficile*-associated disease in chronic renal failure. Am J Med Sci 2000; 319(5): 338-9.
[http://dx.doi.org/10.1016/S0002-9629(15)40762-1] [PMID: 10830559]

[19] Kusumi RK, Plouffe JF, Wyatt RH, Fass RJ. Central nervous system toxicity associated with metronidazole therapy. Ann Intern Med 1980; 93(1): 59-60.
[http://dx.doi.org/10.7326/0003-4819-93-1-59] [PMID: 7396319]

[20] Juillerat P, Pittet V, Felley C, *et al.* Drug safety in Crohn's disease therapy. Digestion 2007; 76(2): 161-8.
[http://dx.doi.org/10.1159/000111031] [PMID: 18239408]

[21] Bonkowsky JL, Sondrup C, Benedict SL. Acute reversible cerebellar lesions associated with metronidazole therapy. Neurology 2007; 68(3): 180.
[http://dx.doi.org/10.1212/01.wnl.0000242579.37851.26] [PMID: 17224569]

[22] Schreiber W, Spernal J. Metronidazole-induced psychotic disorder. Am J Psychiatry 1997; 154(8): 1170-1.
[http://dx.doi.org/10.1176/ajp.154.8.1170b] [PMID: 9247414]

[23] Ahmed A, Loes DJ, Bressler EL. Reversible magnetic resonance imaging findings in metronidazole-induced encephalopathy. Neurology 1995; 45(3 Pt 1): 588-9.
[http://dx.doi.org/10.1212/WNL.45.3.588] [PMID: 7898724]

[24] Woodruff BK, Wijdicks EF, Marshall WF. Reversible metronidazole-induced lesions of the cerebellar dentate nuclei. N Engl J Med 2002; 346(1): 68-9.
[http://dx.doi.org/10.1056/NEJM200201033460117] [PMID: 11778010]

[25] Gerding DN, Muto CA, Owens RC Jr. Treatment of *Clostridium difficile* infection. Clin Infect Dis 2008; 46(1) (Suppl. 1): S32-42.
[http://dx.doi.org/10.1086/521860] [PMID: 18177219]

[26] Castro JA, Diaz de Toranzo EG. Toxic effects of nifurtimox and benznidazole, two drugs used against American trypanosomiasis Chagas disease. Biomed Environ Sci 1988; 1(1): 19-33.
[PMID: 3151755]

[27] Khaw M, Panosian CB. Human antiprotozoal therapy: past, present, and future. Clin Microbiol Rev 1995; 8(3): 427-39.
[PMID: 7553575]

[28] Cui L, Su XZ. Discovery, mechanisms of action and combination therapy of artemisinin. Expert Rev Anti Infect Ther 2009; 7(8): 999-1013.
[http://dx.doi.org/10.1586/eri.09.68] [PMID: 19803708]

[29] Keiser J, Utzinger J. Artemisinins and synthetic trioxolanes in the treatment of helminth infections. Curr Opin Infect Dis 2007; 20(6): 605-12.
[http://dx.doi.org/10.1097/QCO.0b013e3282f19ec4] [PMID: 17975411]

[30] Sen R, Ganguly S, Saha P, Chatterjee M. Efficacy of artemisinin in experimental visceral leishmaniasis. Int J Antimicrob Agents 2010; 36(1): 43-9.
[http://dx.doi.org/10.1016/j.ijantimicag.2010.03.008] [PMID: 20403680]

[31] Mahmoud B, Mahmoud RK, Seyed AK, *et al.* Antiparasitic herbs used in west regions of Ilam province located in west Iran. Asian Pac J Trop Dis 2014; 4(2): S764-9.

[32] Mahmoud B, Seyed AK, Hassan H, Shirin F, *et al.* Ethnobotanic study of medicinal plants in Urmia city: identification and traditional using of anti-parasites plants. Asian Pac J Trop Dis 2014; 4(2): S906-10.

[33] Bolivar P, Cruz-Paredes C, HernAndez LR, *et al.* Antimicrobial, anti-inflammatory, antiparasitic, and cytotoxic activities of *Galium mexicanum.* J Ethnopharmacol 2011; 137(1): 141-7. [http://dx.doi.org/10.1016/j.jep.2011.04.069] [PMID: 21586319]

[34] Bremer Christensen C, Soelberg J, Stensvold Rune C, Jäger AK. Activity of medicinal plants from Ghana against the parasitic gut Blastocystis. J Ethnopharmacol 2015; 174: 569-75.

[35] Tsuyoshi G, Noritaka H, Takaishi Y, Kashiwada Y. Antiparasitic effects of *Sophoraflavescens* root extracts on the ciliate, *Cryptocaryon irritans.* Aquaculture 2015; 435: 173-7. [http://dx.doi.org/10.1016/j.aquaculture.2014.09.007]

[36] Silva AP, Silva MP, Oliveira CG, *et al.* Garcinielliptone FC: antiparasitic activity without cytotoxicity to mammalian cells. Toxicol In Vitro 2015; 29(4): 681-7. [http://dx.doi.org/10.1016/j.tiv.2014.12.014] [PMID: 25553916]

[37] Mai LH, Chabot GG, Grellier P, *et al.* Antivascular and anti-parasite activities of natural and hemisynthetic flavonoids from New Caledonian Gardenia species (Rubiaceae). Eur J Med Chem 2015; 93: 93-100. [http://dx.doi.org/10.1016/j.ejmech.2015.01.012] [PMID: 25659770]

[38] Gontijo VS, Judice WA, Codonho B, *et al.* Leishmanicidal, antiproteolytic and antioxidant evaluation of natural biflavonoids isolated from *Garcinia brasiliensis* and their semisynthetic derivatives. Eur J Med Chem 2012; 58: 613-23. [http://dx.doi.org/10.1016/j.ejmech.2012.06.021] [PMID: 23178961]

[39] Krafts K, Hempelmann E, SkA3rska-Stania A. From methylene blue to chloroquine: a brief review of the development of an antimalarial therapy. Parasitol Res 2012; 111(1): 1-6. [http://dx.doi.org/10.1007/s00436-012-2886-x] [PMID: 22411634]

[40] Abramowicz M, Ed. Drugs for parasitic infections. 1-12.

[41] Nagata N, Marriott D, Harkness J, Ellis JT, Stark D. Current treatment options for Dientamoeba fragilis infections. Int J Parasitol Drugs Drug Resist 2012; 2: 204-15. [http://dx.doi.org/10.1016/j.ijpddr.2012.08.002] [PMID: 24533282]

[42] Pérez-Villanueva J, Romo-Mancillas A, Hernández-Campos A, Yépez-Mulia L, Hernández-Luis F, Castillo R. Antiprotozoal activity of proton-pump inhibitors. Bioorg Med Chem Lett 2011; 21(24): 7351-4. [http://dx.doi.org/10.1016/j.bmcl.2011.10.028] [PMID: 22047694]

[43] LiA ares GE, Ravaschino EL, Rodriguez JB. Progresses in the field of drug design to combat tropical protozoan parasitic diseases. Curr Med Chem 2006; 13(3): 335-60. [http://dx.doi.org/10.2174/092986706775476043] [PMID: 16475941]

[44] Giannini G, Battistuzzi G. Exploring *in vitro* and *in vivo* Hsp90 inhibitors activity against human protozoan parasites. Bioorg Med Chem Lett 2015; 25(3): 462-5.

[http://dx.doi.org/10.1016/j.bmcl.2014.12.048] [PMID: 25547934]

[45] Pandeya SN, Thakkar D. Combinatorial chemistry: a novel method in drug discovery and its application. Indian J Chem 2005; 44B: 335-48.

[46] Geysen HM, Schoenen F, Wagner D, Wagner R. Combinatorial compound libraries for drug discovery: an ongoing challenge. Nat Rev Drug Discov 2003; 2(3): 222-30. [http://dx.doi.org/10.1038/nrd1035] [PMID: 12612648]

[47] Carrol J. Will Combinatorial Chemistry Keep Its Promise? Biotechnol Healthc 2005; 2(3): 26-7. and 31-2

[48] Gamo FJ. Antimalarial drug resistance: new treatments options for *Plasmodium*. Drug Discov Today Technol 2014; 11: 81-8. [http://dx.doi.org/10.1016/j.ddtec.2014.03.002] [PMID: 24847657]

[49] Urbina JA. Chemotherapy of Chagas disease. Curr Pharm Des 2002; 8(4): 287-95. [http://dx.doi.org/10.2174/1381612023396177] [PMID: 11860367]

[50] Elicio PD, Chao MN, Galizzi M, *et al.* Design, synthesis and biological evaluation of WC-9 analogs as antiparasitic agents. Eur J Med Chem 2013; 69: 480-9. [http://dx.doi.org/10.1016/j.ejmech.2013.09.009] [PMID: 24090919]

[51] Matthews KR. 25 years of African trypanosome research: From description to molecular dissection and new drug discovery. Mol Biochem Parasitol 2015; 200(1-2): 30-40.

[52] Stolfa DA, Marek M, Lancelot J, *et al.* Molecular basis for the antiparasitic activity of a mercaptoacetamide derivative that inhibits histone deacetylase 8 (HDAC8) from the human pathogen *schistosoma mansoni.* J Mol Biol 2014; 426(20): 3442-53. [http://dx.doi.org/10.1016/j.jmb.2014.03.007] [PMID: 24657767]

[53] Chaal BK, Gupta AP, Wastuwidyaningtyas BD, Luah YH, Bozdech Z. Histone deacetylases play a major role in the transcriptional regulation of the Plasmodium falciparum life cycle. PLoS Pathog 2010. retrieved from: http://www.ncbi.nlm.nih.gov/pubmed/20107518.

[54] Shibi IG, Aswathy L, Jisha RS, Masand VH, Divyachandran A, Gajbhiye JM. Molecular docking and QSAR analyses for understanding the antimalarial activity of some 7-substituted-4-aminoquinoline derivatives. Eur J Pharm Sci 2015; 77: 9-23. [http://dx.doi.org/10.1016/j.ejps.2015.05.025] [PMID: 26006759]

[55] Scalese G, Benítez J, Rostán S, *et al.* Expanding the family of heteroleptic oxidovanadium(IV) compounds with salicylaldehyde semicarbazones and polypyridyl ligands showing anti-Trypanosoma cruzi activity. J Inorg Biochem 2015; 147: 116-25.

[56] Flannery EL, Chatterjee AK, Winzeler EA. Antimalarial drug discovery - approaches and progress towards new medicines. Nat Rev Microbiol 2013; 11(12): 849-62. [http://dx.doi.org/10.1038/nrmicro3138] [PMID: 24217412]

[57] Graz B, Willcox ML, Diakite C, *et al.* Argemone mexicana decoction *versus* artesunate-amodiaquine for the management of malaria in Mali: policy and public-health implications. Trans R Soc Trop Med Hyg 2010; 104(1): 33-41. [http://dx.doi.org/10.1016/j.trstmh.2009.07.005] [PMID: 19733875]

[58] Chang YC, Chang FR, Khalil AT, Hsieh PW, Wu YC. Cytotoxic benzophenanthridine and benzylisoquinoline alkaloids from Argemone mexicana. Z Naturforsch, C, J Biosci 2003; 58(7-8): 521-6.
[http://dx.doi.org/10.1515/znc-2003-7-813] [PMID: 12939038]

[59] Mesia K, Tona L, Mampunza MM, *et al.* Antimalarial efficacy of a quantified extract of Nauclea pobeguinii stem bark in human adult volunteers with diagnosed uncomplicated falciparum malaria. Part 2: a clinical phase IIB trial. Planta Med 2012; 78(9): 853-60.
[http://dx.doi.org/10.1055/s-0031-1298488] [PMID: 22538476]

[60] Rottmann M, McNamara C, Yeung BK, *et al.* Spiroindolones, a potent compound class for the treatment of malaria. Science 2010; 329(5996): 1175-80.
[http://dx.doi.org/10.1126/science.1193225] [PMID: 20813948]

[61] Yeung BK, Zou B, Rottmann M, *et al.* Spirotetrahydro beta-carbolines (spiroindolones): a new class of potent and orally efficacious compounds for the treatment of malaria. J Med Chem 2010; 53(14): 5155-64.
[http://dx.doi.org/10.1021/jm100410f] [PMID: 20568778]

[62] Wu T, Nagle A, Kuhen K, *et al.* Imidazolopiperazines: hit to lead optimization of new antimalarial agents. J Med Chem 2011; 54(14): 5116-30.
[http://dx.doi.org/10.1021/jm2003359] [PMID: 21644570]

[63] Charman SA, Arbe-Barnes S, Bathurst IC, *et al.* Synthetic ozonide drug candidate OZ439 offers new hope for a single-dose cure of uncomplicated malaria. Proc Natl Acad Sci USA 2011; 108(11): 4400-5.
[http://dx.doi.org/10.1073/pnas.1015762108] [PMID: 21300861]

[64] Nilsen A, LaCrue AN, White KL, *et al.* Quinolone-3-diarylethers: a new class of antimalarial drug. Sci Transl Med 2013; 5(177): 177ra37.
[http://dx.doi.org/10.1126/scitranslmed.3005029] [PMID: 23515079]

[65] Brun R, Blum J, Chappuis F, Burri C. Human African trypanosomiasis. Lancet 2010; 375(9709): 148-59.
[http://dx.doi.org/10.1016/S0140-6736(09)60829-1] [PMID: 19833383]

[66] Mäser P, Wittlin S, Rottmann M, Wenzler T, Kaiser M, Brun R. Antiparasitic agents: new drugs on the horizon. Curr Opin Pharmacol 2012; 12(5): 562-6.
[http://dx.doi.org/10.1016/j.coph.2012.05.001] [PMID: 22652215]

[67] a) Avialable at: www.dndi.org/diseases-projects/portfolio/fexinidazole.html.. ; b) Tarral A, Blesson S, Mordt OV, *et al.* Determination of an optimal dosing regimen for fexinidazole, a novel oral drug for the treatment of human African trypanosomiasis: first-in-human studies. Clin Pharmacokinet 2014; 53(6): 565-80.
[http://dx.doi.org/10.1007/s40262-014-0136-3] [PMID: 24535888]

[68] a) Avialable at: http://www.dndi.org/diseases-projects/portfolio/oxaborole-scyx-7158.html.. ; b) Jacobs RT, Nare B, Wring SA, *et al.* SCYX-7158, an orally-active benzoxaborole for the treatment of stage 2 human African trypanosomiasis. PLoS Negl Trop Dis 2011; 5(6): e1151.
[http://dx.doi.org/10.1371/journal.pntd.0001151] [PMID: 21738803]

[69] Avialable at: http://www.cdc.gov/parasites/leishmaniasis/health_professionals/index.html#tx..

[70] Avialable at: http://whqlibdoc.who.int/hq/2011/a95053_eng.pdf..

[71] Mossallam SF, Amer EI, El-Faham MH. Efficacy of SynriamTM, a new antimalarial combination of OZ277 and piperaquine, against different developmental stages of Schistosoma mansoni. Acta Trop 2015; 143: 36-46.
[http://dx.doi.org/10.1016/j.actatropica.2014.12.005] [PMID: 25530543]

[72] Moraes CB, Giardini MA, Kim H, *et al.* Nitroheterocyclic compounds are more efficacious than CYP51 inhibitors against *Trypanosoma cruzi*: implications for Chagas disease drug discovery and development. Sci Rep 2014; 4: 4703.
[http://dx.doi.org/10.1038/srep04703] [PMID: 24736467]

[73] Buckner FS, Urbina JA. Recent developments in sterol 14-demethylase inhibitors for Chagas disease. Int J Parasitol Drugs Drug Resist 2012; 2: 236-42.
[http://dx.doi.org/10.1016/j.ijpddr.2011.12.002] [PMID: 23277882]

[74] Avialable at: http://www.dndi.org/diseases-projects/portfolio/azoles-e1224.html

CHAPTER 3

Crude Extracts and Isolated Compounds with Trypanocidal Activity

Paz M. Salazar Schettino[*], **Gloria Rojas**, **Margarita Cabrera** and **Martha Bucio**

Laboratorio de Biología de Parásitos, Departamento de Microbiología y Parasitología, Facultad de Medicina, Universidad Nacional Autónoma de México, Mexico City, 04510, Mexico

Abstract: Chagas' disease, or American trypanosomiasis, is a potentially mortal disease caused by the protozoan *Trypanosoma cruzi*. It is included in the list of neglected diseases or poverty-linked diseases. An estimate of 5.7 million people in the endemic areas are infected, resulting in 7000 yearly deaths. The disease is distributed in Central and South America, Mexico, and the southern United States. Due to rural-urban migration, the parasite is transmitted by blood transfusion, by vertical transmission from mother to child, or by organ transplantation; on the other side, some cases have been detected in non-endemic zones both in America and in Europe. Chagas' disease is among the 17 neglected diseases; it is a complex zoonosis, involving interaction of vectors species with wild, peridomestic, and domestic mammals, showing several clinical pictures and transmission modes. It poses the highest economic burden among parasitic diseases in Latin America due to its long chronicity. The clinical manifestations and epidemiologic traits of the disease vary from region to region. The current medication against *T. cruzi*, nifurtimox and benznidazole, has adverse effects. Aiming to make new treatment alternatives known, the activity of plant-isolated compounds from Central America, South America, and Mexico is herein discussed, along with their action against different stages of *Trypanosoma cruzi*.

Keywords: Chagas disease, Crude extracts, Medicinal plants, *Trypanosoma cruzi*.

[*] **Corresponding author Paz M. Salazar Schettino:** Laboratorio de Biología de Parásitos, Departamento de Microbiología y Parasitología, Facultad de Medicina, Universidad Nacional Autónoma de México, Mexico City, 04510, Mexico; Tel: (52) 5556232381; E-mail: pazmar@unam.mx

Norma Rivera (Ed.)

INTRODUCTION

Chagas' disease, or American trypanosomiasis, is a potentially mortal disease caused by the protozoan parasite *Trypanosoma cruzi* and transmitted by hematophagous hemipterans of the Reduviidae family. It is included in the list of neglected diseases or poverty-linked diseases. An estimate of 5.7 million people are infected in the endemic areas, which includes the 21 countries in Latin America, resulting in 7000 yearly deaths and over 70 million are at risk for becoming infected. The disease is distributed in Central and South America, Mexico, and the southern United States [1 - 5]. Rural-to-urban migration in Latin America during the 1970s and 1980s changed the epidemiologic patterns of the disease, turning it into an urban infection where the parasite can be transmitted without a vector [3]. Due to an increase in population movements, the number of diagnosed cases increased even in non-endemic countries both in America and in Europe. A 2011 study reported between 68,000 and 122,000 cases in European countries [6]; this increase poses additional risks for parasite transmission by blood transfusion, vertical transmission from mother to child, or organ transplantation [7 - 9]. Currently regarded as a public health issue in several countries of the Americas, the World Health Organization/Pan American Health Organization (WHO/PAHO) place Chagas' disease among the 17 priority neglected diseases [10 - 12].

The disease was discovered in 1909 by Carlos Chagas, in Brazil. The acute form of Chagas' disease was first described in Berenice, a 2-year-old girl who died at age 82 from other causes. Although infected, she did not acquire the disease. Chagas also described the morphology and the life cycle of the parasite in vertebrate hosts and in vectors insects, and made observations on the course of infection in laboratory animals and in cultures. This clinical entity is a complex zoonosis, with recurrent infections involving the interaction of vectors species with wild, peridomestic, and domestic mammals, showing several clinical pictures and transmission modes. It poses the highest economic burden among parasitic diseases in Latin America due to its long chronicity. Since 1909, Carlos Chagas refers to the rural housing conditions as posing risk or promoting vector propagation, and these conditions are still prevalent nowadays [13]. The clinical manifestations and epidemiologic traits of the disease vary from region to region.

Biology of Chagas' Disease

Trypanosoma cruzi is a flagellate protozoan of the phylum Sarcomastigophora, order Kinetoplastida, and family Trypanosomatidae. The parasite goes through three main developmental stages: trypomastigote (bloodborne when it is in the bloodstream of its mammal host, and metacyclic in the feces of vectors), epimastigote in the intestine of the triatomine and in culture media, and amastigote when located inside the cells of the mammal host. The trypomastigote stage shows a 10-20 μm elongated body, vesicular nucleus, slightly granular cytoplasm, and a terminal kinetoplast with diffuse chromatin from which the membrane emerges. Epimastigote is fusiform and can be up to 30-μm long; kinetoplast has a chromatin organized in a compact manner at the anterior portion, near the nucleus; the parasite has a flagellum and an undulating membrane. Amastigote does not exhibit an external flagellum, but nucleus and kinetoplast are visible; the cell, 3-5 μm in diameter, is a multiplication or fission form inside host cells [14 - 17]. Both vectors arthropods and humans play a role in *T. cruzi* life cycle, along with a large number of reservoir mammals, mainly possums, armadillos, squirrels, field mice, rats, donkeys, pigs, dogs, and cats [18].

Vectors insects carry the infective forms (metacyclic trypomastigotes) of *T. cruzi* in feces, which are deposited on the skin during or after feeding; after entering the host through skin or mucosa, the parasite is able to invade a wide variety of cells where it transforms into the amastigote stage, a replicative intracellular form. Eventually, amastigotes will give rise to trypomastigote forms, which disseminate to other cells and can be ingested by the vector. When a triatomine ingests blood from an infected mammal, the parasite enters the bug; epimastigotes develop in the intestine lumen of the insect, multiplying by binary fission, and about 15-30 days later the metacyclic trypomastigote stage, the infective form, is produced and expelled with the feces of triatomines. When a parasite-infected triatomine feeds again on a healthy mammal, its stomach fills to repletion and discharges feces containing metacyclic trypomastigotes (Fig. **1**).

Trypanosoma cruzi has a wide array of surface molecules that allow it to make contact with mammal cells and complete the infection process. Membrane molecules start a host-parasite signaling process; among these, lipid rafts in parasite member regulate membrane fluidity, favoring invasion to mammal cells [19].

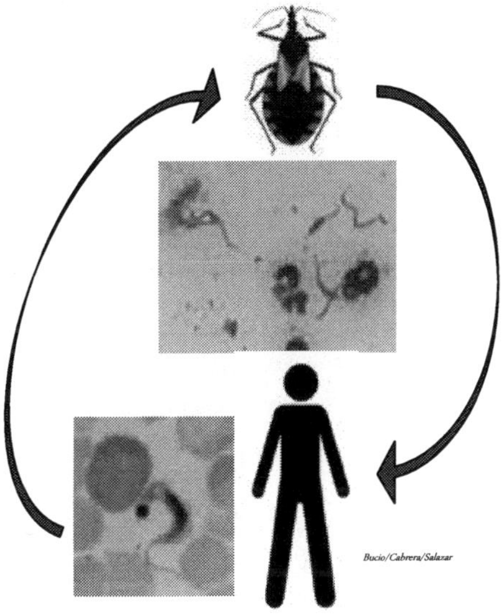

Fig. (1). Life cycle of *Trypanosoma cruzi.*

Trans-sialidases could be related to the host cell invasion process, protecting the parasite from the host immune response [20].

Mucins are a group of surface glycoproteins in *T. cruzi.* Sugar residues in those molecules interact with mammal and vector cells, and their role could be either to protect the parasite from vector or host defensive mechanisms or to ensure the invasion of specific cells or tissues [21, 22].

The gp82, gp35, and gp50 glycoproteins, molecules expressed on the surface of metacyclic trypomastigotes, are related to parasite invasion by inducing an increase in intracellular calcium both in parasite and host cells [23, 24].

Gp90 is a surface glycoprotein present in *T. cruzi* metacyclic trypomastigotes, acting as a negative regulator of cell invasion since it does not trigger calcium signaling, even though it is known to show glycosidase and anti-phagocytic activity [21, 23].

Other proteins involved in the parasite interaction with mammal cells are gp83, related to protein kinase C (PKC) in macrophages; penetrin; cruzipain, an endoprotease found in the four main parasite stages; oligopeptidase B, a serine-endoprotease involved in the increased calcium transit in host cells; and Tc80, a collagenase related with extracellular matrix degradation in host tissues, thus facilitating invasion [23, 25 - 27].

Based on molecular studies, several genetic polymorphisms have been determined in different *T. cruzi* populations. Currently, the parasite is classified into six discrete typifying units, labeled Tc I to Tc VI. Tc I has been found from Argentina through the United States, while Tc II-VI are distributed from the Amazon basin to southern Argentina. However, there exist places where all discrete typifying units are present; this is the case of Colombia, where Tc I has been reported as predominant while Tc II, Tc III, Tc IV, and Tc VI are found in lower proportion [28 - 30].

Vectors

All *T. cruzi* vectors are hematophagous insects from the phylum Arthropoda, subphylum Hexapoda, order Hemiptera, family Reduviidae, and subfamily Triatominae [31]. Subfamily Triatominae is composed by 5 tribes and 15 genera; 140 species are known. About 125 species in this family are found in the Americas, between 42° N latitude, southern United States, and 42° S latitude, southern Argentina. They survive in 30-60% humidity conditions, temperature of 24-28 °C [31 - 35], and altitude ranging between 10 and 1500 meters above sea level [36].

They are obligate hematophagous, hemimetabolous insects, with five nymph stages and an adult stage, all of which are capable of transmitting *T. cruzi* [8, 33, 37].

A wide diversity of transmitter bugs, with 32 different species, has been described in Mexico. From these, 19 species belong to the genus *Triatoma,* six to the genus *Meccus,* two to the genus *Panstrongylus*, and one to each of the genera *Belminus, Dipetalogaster*, *Eratyrus, Paratriatoma,* and *Rhodnius* [38, 39].

Only those arthropod species adapted to the human environment are epidemiologically linked to Chagas' disease. Their distribution has reduced after the control programs undertaken as part of the Initiatives of the Southern Cone, programs of the Andean countries and of Central American countries [5, 40].

Trypanosoma cruzi in the Vectors

When the vector ingests blood from an infected host, it stores it in its stomach, where digestion begins immediately. Some bloodborne trypomastigotes are lysed and some other start differentiating into epimastigotes. Then they pass into the Malpighi's tubules and the posterior midgut, where epimastigotes bind the perimicrovillar membrane (PMM) through glycoconjugate formation, and divide by longitudinal binary fission [21, 41].

It has been described that 1-2 weeks later, epimastigotes in the surface of rectal epithelium differentiate into metacyclic trypomastigotes, the infective form, and are discharged in feces [41].

The association of the parasite with the digestive tract epithelium is different in the vector midgut and the hindgut. In the posterior midgut, epimastigotes are in contact with PMM, and in the rectum they are bound by hydrophobic or lectin interactions [41, 42]. The binding of *T. cruzi* to glycoproteins in the vector gut has been proposed as a signal to begin epimastigote differentiation into metacyclic trypomastigotes [43, 44].

Natural History of the Disease

The natural history of Chagas' disease is that of a systemic, chronic parasitic infection, which can lead to severe cardiopathy forms or mega-, usually digestive deformations. In general, control programs have focused funds and strategies on eradicating those insects more closely associated to the human habitat, relegating the infected patient to the background. With regard to case detection, only those cases with concrete pathologies are reported, thus overshadowing all other cases (over 70%) of persons infected by *T. cruzi* but with no apparent manifestations; this minimizes the perception on the actual magnitude of the disease [45].

Control strategies for Chagas' disease are based on interrupting vector transmission; on a systematic blood screening from donors from affected countries; on detection and treatment of mother-to-child transmission, and on treatment administration to acute cases and children. Available figures are controversial with regard to the incidence and prevalence of the infection and the disease and with regard to what fraction of infected patients will develop the disease. In some regions of Latin America, Chagas' disease is the main cause of cardiac-related death among young adults.

Some improvement has been achieved by interrupting vector transmission in the whole territory or in certain regions of the affected countries, by requiring a universal screening of blood donors, by extending the coverage of diagnostics and access to treatment, by improving the quality of diagnostics, clinical care, and treatment for infected and affected individuals. While substantial progress has been made, not all countries have met the proposed goals, and new challenges are emerging [40].

Currently, two phases of the disease are described: acute and chronic; the latter can be either symptomatic chronic or asymptomatic chronic (previously known as indeterminate phase), depending on the presence of characteristic symptoms and signs. Clinical findings in the acute phase are related to the parasite entry site, causing a local inflammatory reaction with acute regional lymphadenitis; this primary complex is observed after a short incubation period (7 days) and lasts about one month. Trypomastigotes are found in peripheral blood and cerebrospinal fluid of patients with acute infection. When the parasite enters through the ocular conjunctive, Romaña's sign (unilateral bipalpebral edema) with preauricular lymphadenitis (primary complex) is observed (Fig. **2**). If the parasite enters through the skin, the lesion will appear as a pruritic, reddish- or violet-colored nodule, with regional ganglia enlargement (inoculation chagoma). Most individuals are asymptomatic or show unspecific manifestations; however, children, elderly persons, and less frequently adults may develop severe symptoms after the incubation period. The main systemic manifestations are fever, tachycardia, lymphadenopathy, hepatosplenomegaly, nausea, vomiting, anorexia, and edema. About 1% of acute phase patients die from complications associated to acute myocarditis or meningoencephalitis. Most acute phase patients recover satisfactorily in a 3-4 weeks period. Diagnostic is established by parasite identification in blood smear or thick drop examination, and by microhematocrit.

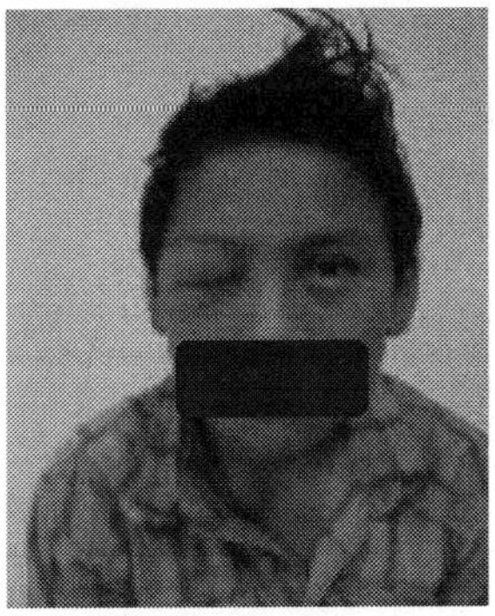

Fig. (2). Romaña sign in patient with acute Chagas disease.

The asymptomatic chronic phase is a long period of clinical silence after parasite primary infection; its duration is variable, from years to decades and even a lifetime; patients show scanty parasitemia due to the parasite slow intracellular multiplication, and show antibodies elicited by the multiple antigens in *T. cruzi.* Serological techniques are the methods of choice for diagnosis, and due to the low parasitemia, occasionally xenodiagnostic or hemoculture. The importance of this phase lies in that asymptomatic infected individuals pose a high risk of transfusional transmission in blood banks and mother-to-child (connatal) transmission.

Among those patients progressing to the symptomatic chronic phase, 27% show manifestations related to cardiac lesions, 6% digestive lesions (megacolon or megaesophagus), and 3% a compromised peripheral nervous system [46]. The methods of choice for diagnosis in this phase are serologic tests and radiologic or imaging studies. The progression from asymptomatic Chagas' disease to chronic cardiomyopathy is still controversial, and several hypotheses have been proposed correlating histopathological lesions directly produced by the presence of the parasite with the ensuing chronic inflammatory process, by autoimmunity mechanisms, and by toxin-triggered lesions. The mega- pathogeny is mainly related with a destruction of mesenteric nervous plexuses. In extreme cases, these pathologies can cause death (Fig. **3**).

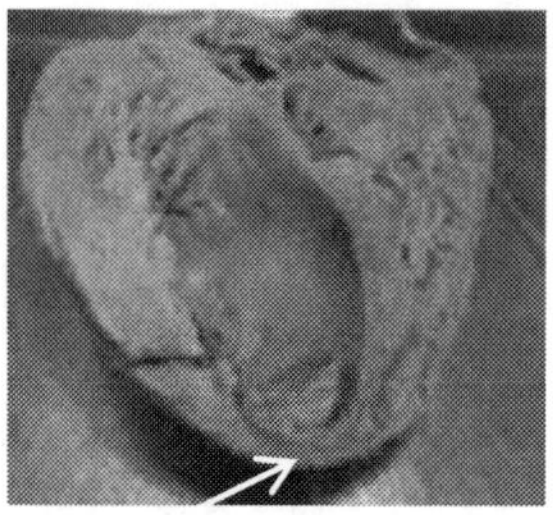

Fig. (3). Sagittal cut heart in a case with chronic Chagas disease. Fibrosis is noted in apical region.

Pathogenesis of Chronic Cardiomyopathy

The main lesions in Chagas' disease are found in the autonomous nervous system and in myocardium. This immunopathogenic process is very complex. After infection and lysis of myocardial cells, a specific immune reaction against *T. cruzi* is elicited, with activation of phagocytic and cytotoxic cells and production of Th1-type cytokines (IL-1, IFN-γ, and TNF-α) to activate and recruit monocytes to the infection site; as a result, a control of parasite replication is established. Phagocytic cells are activated by interferon gamma (IFN-γ), the main cytokine involved in this process. While this Th1 response protects the host during the acute phase, in chronicity it is associated to myocardial damage by an exacerbated inflammatory response, chiefly with TCD8+ lymphocytes and IFN-γ production; the latter induces nitric oxide production in macrophages, which in turn leads to myocardial lesion and damage to nervous fibers by oxidative stress [47 - 49].

The damage to heart and intestinal tract tissues in the acute phase is directly related to parasitemia and tissue parasitism. The characteristic lesion in chronic cardiopathy, on the other hand, is a diffuse myocarditis with lymphocytic infiltrates; there is presence of immunoglobulins, scanty parasitic elements, and small inflammatory focuses that produce myocellular hypertrophy, myocytolysis, and intense reparative fibrosis with interstitial accumulation of collagen fibers; this leads to ventricular remodeling and function deterioration, first diastolic and then systolic. The cytokines involved in this process are profibrotic, primarily TGF-β, along with TNF-α, MIP-1α, IL-8, IL-13, and IFN-γ; the ensuing fibrosis impairs cavitary motility with heart function deterioration [50].

Since the 1950's, Köberle enriched the histopathology of the disease by describing the parasitism associated to an intense cardiac neuronal depopulation, periganglionitis, and degenerative changes in Schwann cells and nervous fibers; he also standardized the technique of neuronal counting in the heart and in the autonomous nervous system at organs with ganglion damage [51]. Parasympathetic periganglionic inflammation with adhesion of inflammatory mononuclear cells to neurons leads to lysis; added to the autoimmune neuronal reaction, it induces the characteristic autonomic dysfunction, which could be detected before the development of ventricular dysfunction in all disease phases, even in the asymptomatic and digestive forms. These neurogenic alterations in the chronic phase may cause sudden death, as well as malignant arrhythmias by parasympathetic denervation; on the other hand, the presence and progression of dyssynergic areas in both ventricles lead to a depression of the global ventricular function; finally, mitral and tricuspid insufficiency due to cardiomegaly is observed [52, 53].

There are also microvascular anomalies that lead to myocardial ischemia by two mechanisms that increase the adhesion of platelets to the microvascular endothelium: the inflammatory process with proliferation at the intima and endothelin increase, and neuraminidase production by trypomastigotes. The presence of different-staged thrombi is frequent in the left ventricle and in the right auricle; it is associated to pulmonary, cerebral, spleen, and kidney thrombosis, and it is a common cause of death in chronic cardiopaths [35, 52, 54].

With regard to the autoimmunity observed in this pathology, Torres pointed out in 1941 that a repeated *T. cruzi* infection produces a status he called "allergic", characterized by diffuse infiltrates with macrophages, plasmatic cells, and lymphocytes, along with connective tissue proliferation even in the absence of the parasite, corresponding to a late hypersensitivity response (Type IV) [55]. It has been demonstrated that over 80% of cases in this cardiomyopathy exhibit autoreactive antibodies against various tissues, tissular structures, cells, and even against β-adrenergic and muscarinic receptors [56 - 58].

This chronic phase has been described in adults, and it is worthy to mention that there is no information in the literature about this stage in children.

Laboratory Diagnostics

The first serological test to diagnose *T. cruzi* infection was the Guerreiro and Machado reaction in 1913; it consisted of a complement fixation assay [59]; Boyden used the indirect hemagglutination test for the first time in 1951, with good results [60]; Camargo standardized the indirect immunofluorescence technique in 1966 [61], and Voller used the indirect ELISA technique in microplate in 1975 [62].

The presence of parasites and anti-*Trypanosoma cruzi* antibodies are the most relevant elements for laboratory diagnostics. Parasitological diagnosis is usually made during the acute infection phase, which is very short with respect to the other phase. Serological tests are aimed to detect and confirm infected or ill individuals, and they are useful tools to evaluate therapeutic measures and to monitor sanitary programs. Serological tests are devised according to two criteria: When an easy and rapid detection of infected or ill individuals is required (screening), a high sensitivity is mandatory even though specificity is lower; or when case confirmation is required either after showing reactivity in screening tests or when clinical and/or epidemiological data are compatible with the disease. These tests are called confirmatory, and must show high specificity and sensitivity; WHO/PAHO recommends using ELISA, IFI, or HAI as routine, conventional methods, and recombinant antigens and PCR (polymerase chain-reaction) as non-conventional methods, the latter still having limitations for massive use.

Desk Studies

The first used desk studies, still in use to date, are radiologic; diverse degrees of cardiac dilation (cardiomegaly) or of cavities with left ventricle enlargement, biventricular enlargement, and pulmonary vascular congestion can be detected by radiologic studies. Experience showed the existence of cardiopathies where cardiac silhouettes within normal limits were observed. Therefore, the use of electrocardiography (ECG) is recommended whenever possible; in this cardiopathy, ECG shows alterations according to the evolutionary stage. In the acute phase, records are generally unspecific. In the chronic phase, ECG records can show data of left ventricle enlargement. ECG alterations could suggest the diagnostic of chagasic cardiomyopathy; however, epidemiological, serological, and clinical data should always be taken into account. In echocardiography, a dilation cardiomyopathy with anomalies in parietal motility, hypertrophy, thinning, or even apical aneurysm (pathognomonic sign) are observed [63]

Therapeutic Management of the Infection and Disease

Currently, nifurtimox (4[(5-nitrofurfurylidene)amino]-3-methylthiomorpholine-1, 1-didioxide) (1972) and benznidazole (N-benzyl-2-nitroimidazole-1 acetamide) (1974) constitute the specific chemotherapy against *T. cruzi;* both drugs were initially used for the acute phase and later in the chronic phase of the disease, especially in the child and young population. Now, the priority in research is on developing new drugs that offer shorter treatment times and less adverse reactions. Clinical assays have demonstrated that the treatment has an efficacy over 60% in the early chronic phase (children under the age of 15), using serological and parasitological tests as criteria of cure. However, adverse effects have been reported for both drugs, such as malaise and digestive alterations: weight loss, gastric distress, nausea, and vomiting; hematologic alterations (due to hypersensitivity): leucopenia, thrombocytopenia, agranulocytosis; dermatologic alterations: erythema and atopic dermatitis (mild or severe); and neurological alterations such as dose-dependent polyneuropathies [64, 65].

In 2013, DNDi reported the development of a new pediatric dosage form of benznidazole. The treatment was registered in Brazil (2011) and it was included in the WHO List of Essential Medicines for children in 2013 [66].

Due to the adverse effects of the two drugs currently used to treat Chagas' disease, there is an urgent need of new therapeutic options; a literature review shows a wide array of studies focused on researching new antitrypanosomal drugs, as well as biologic research on the anti-*T. cruzi* effects of plants, chiefly from Central and South America. The WHO has promoted the study of plants used in traditional medicine; thus, four compendia were published between 1999 and 2009, which included 117 monographies describing quality assurance and use of selected medicinal plants. In contrast with the large number of medicinal plants used against *Plasmodium falciparum,* for instance, only two medicinal plants with anti-*T. cruzi* activity are reported [67]. Table **1** shows the studies aimed to research plants showing action *in vitro* against the main stages of *T. cruzi* [67 - 91] In this context, *in silico* phytochemical studies of plants that have shown activity against *T. cruzi* are also valuable [92, 93].

Table 1. Plants with anti *Trypanosoma cruzi* activity.

Scientific name	Family	Material of interest	Geographical distribution	Studied chemical composition	Trypanocidal activity
Rosmarinus officinalis L.	Lamiaceae	Leaves	Cultivated worldwide	Two triterpenic acids: oleanolic and ursolic	Inhibition of *T. cruzi* epimastigote motility after 2 h incubation, at 2.0 mg/ml [67]
Neurolaena lobata	Asteraceae	Leaves	Guatemala	Sesquiterpene lactones	Fraction 2. IC90 25.6 and 125.4 µg/ml on trypomastigotes and epimastigotes, respectively, isolated from human-borne *T. cruzi* [68]
Mikania cordifolia	Asteraceae	Leaves		Butanolic fraction	Inhibition of *T. cruzi* Y strain epimastigote proliferation close to 100% [69]
Polygala sabulosa *Polygala paniculata*	Polygalaceae	Aerial parts	Brazil	Styrilpyrones and prenylcoumarines. Dichloromethane and hexane fractions	LD50 of 5-10 µg/ml on epimastigotes. 100% trypomastigote Y strain reduction [70]
Camellia sinenesis	Theaceae	Leaves	China	Fraction 5 Polyphenolic compounds. Catechins	50% lytic activity on trypomastigotes at 0.12-85 pM and 50% growth inhibition on Tulahuen strain amastigotes at 100 nM [71]

(Table 1) contd.....

Scientific name	Family	Material of interest	Geographical distribution	Studied chemical composition	Trypanocidal activity
Piper cumanense	Piperaceae	Leaves, bark	Colombia	Ethanolic extract	IC_{50} (µg/ml) < 12.5 on Tulahuen strain epimastigotes
Acnistus arborescens	Solanaceae	Aerial parts	Colombia, Costa Rica, Mexico, Brazil	Ethanolic extract	IC_{50} (µg/ml) < 12.5 on Tulahuen strain epimastigotes [72]
Moquinia kingii	Asteraceae	Aerial parts	Brazil	Flavonoid and sesquiterpene lactone (chloroform crude extract), apigenin and cynaropicrin	IC_{50} values for trypanocidal activity for cynaropicrin and apigenin were 93.5 µg/ml and 181 µg/ml, respectively. *T. cruzi* Y strain [73]
Xilopia aromatica	Annonaceae	Seeds	Colombia	Acetogenins	70% epimastigote mortality with 211.6 µg/ml [74]
Cimbopogon citratus	Poaceae / Gramineae	Leaves	Asia, Africa, Australia	Geranial and neral (citral isomers)	IC_{50} = 126.5 µg/ml, ultrastructural alterations in epimastigotes. Trypomastigote lysis with 50 µg/ml and amastigote lysis with 5 µg/ml at 48 h [75]
Origanum vulgare L.	Labiatae	Aerial parts	Brazil	3-cyclohexen-1-ol	Crude extract of oregano essential oil inhibited epimastigote growth (IC_{50}/24h = 175 µg/ml) and also induced trypomastigote lysis (IC_{50}/24h = 115 µg/ml) [76]

(Table 1) contd.....

Scientific name	Family	Material of interest	Geographical distribution	Studied chemical composition	Trypanocidal activity
Thymus vulgaris L.	Labiatae	Aerial parts	Brazil	Thymol	Thyme essential oil presented IC_{50}/24h values of 77 μg/ml on epimastigotes and 38 μg/ml on trypomastigotes, while treatment with thymol yielded an IC_{50}/24h of 62 μg/ml on epimastigotes and 53 μg/ml on trypomastigotes [76]
Syzygium aromaticum	Myrtaceae	Oil	Brazil	Eugenol	IC_{50} = 99.5 μg/ml on epimastigotes and 57.5μg/ml on trypomastigotes. Ultrastructural alterations, mainly in the nucleus on *T. cruzi* Y strain [77]
Cimbopogon citratus	Poaceae / Gramineae	Essencial oil		Citral	IC_{50} = 30.8 μg/ml Inhibited metacyclogenesis at 24 h. Morphologic alterations in epimastigotes [78]
Aloysia triphylla	Verbenaceae	Leaves	South America	Citral (geranial and neral mixture)	IC_{50} < 100 μg/ml inhibitory activity on *T. cruzi* epimastigotes [79]
Hieronyma antioquensis	Euphorbiaceae	Whole plant	Colombia	n/d	IC_{50} = 3.125, 11.48, and 2.85 μg/ml on epimastigotes, trypomastigotes, and amastigotes, respectively [80]

(Table 1) contd.....

Scientific name	Family	Material of interest	Geographical distribution	Studied chemical composition	Trypanocidal activity
Baccharis retusa	Asteraceae	Leaves	Brazil	Flavanones	Against *T. cruzi* Y strain trypomastigotes (IC_{50} = 20.17 µg/ml). 100% parasites eliminated [81]
Cimbopogon citratus	Poaceae / Gramineae	Leaves	Peru	Citral	Reduction in parasitemia, number of amastigote nests and inflammatory infiltrates in Balb/c mouse heart [82]
Lippia sidoidesL. origanoides	Verbenaceae		Brazil	Monoterpenes and sesquiterpenes	IC_{50} = 28.9 and 10.3 µg/ml on epimastigotes and trypomastigotes, respectively [83]
Zanthoxylum chiloperone	Rutaceae	Leaves	Paraguay		Variable trypanocidal activity on 10 *T. cruzi* strains [84]
Piper ovatum	Piperaceae	Leaves	Brazil	Amide: piperovatine and piperlonguminine	Dose-dependent activity of piperovatine and piperlonguminine: IC_{50} = 41.5 and 53.8 µg/ml, respectively, on epimastigotes; IC_{50} = 35 and 33.9 µg/ml on Y strain amastigotes. Alterations in amastigote mitochondrion and plasmatic membrane [85]
Miconia spp	Melastomataceae	n/d	South America, Mexico	Triterpenes: ursolic and Oleanolic acids	Significant trypanocidal activity of species from genus *Miconia* [86]

(Table 1) contd.....

Scientific name	Family	Material of interest	Geographical distribution	Studied chemical composition	Trypanocidal activity
Casearia sylvestris	Salicaceae	Leaves	Brazil	Casearins	Alteration in plasma membrane permeability of *T. cruzi* Y strain trypomastigotes [87]
10 plants from Mexico	Asteraceae; Simarubaceae; Poaceae; Apiaceae; Fabaceae; Verbenaceae; Lamiaceae; Lauraceae; Rutaceae; Anacardiaceae	Leaves, bark and aerial parts	Peru, Mexico	Terpenes, flavonoids, citral, furanocoumarins, and quinolone alkaloids, among others	88-100% growth inhibition on CL Brener strain epimastigotes at 150 μg/ml [88].
Cinnamomun verum	Lauraceae	bark		Cinnamaldehyde and eugenol	Acción en la cepa Dm28c En epimastigotes= IC_{50} 24.13 μg/ml. Tripomastigotes: IC_{50}=5.05 μg/ml y amastigotes: IC_{50}=20 μg/ml [89]
Pilocarpus spicatus	Rutaceae	Roots, stems, and leaves	Southern Mexico, Central America, Southern South America	Tridecanone, 2-heptadecanone, spathulenol, aromadendrene, β-caryophyllene, 3α-hydroxytirucall--7,24-dien-21-oic acid, (+)-isoangenomaline, episesamin, and sesamin	Growth inhibition on Y strain epimastigotes: 79% with leaf hexane extract, 56% with leaf methanolic extract, and 62% with root methanolic extract [90]
Artemisia absinthium L.	Compositae (Asteraceae)	Flowers	Spain	*trans*-caryophyllene	99.4% growth inhibition at 100 μg/ml on Y strain epimastigotes [91]

CONCLUDING REMARKS

A review on new approaches for the treatment of Chagas' disease results in the finding of compounds derived from natural products that have been used for centuries to treat several diseases, especially in tropical or subtropical regions of developing countries. Being affordable for the general population, medicinal plants are important resources in these countries.

The action of the natural products specifically studied as potential drugs to treat Chagas' disease has been assessed in epimastigotes, trypomastigotes, and amastigotes, as well as their action in metacyclogenesis and cytotoxicity in cell cultures. *In silico* research is another approach to hint the interactions of several phytochemical agents with a known trypanocidal activity with the cell system of *T. cruzi.* While extensive research on new drug design and on the isolation of natural-source compounds is ongoing, the current treatment still relies on nifurtimox and benznidazole.

CONFLICT OF INTEREST

The authors confirm that they have no conflict of interest to declare for this publication.

ACKNOWLEDGEMENTS

Declared none.

GLOSSARY

Benznidazole = (N-benzyl-2-nitroimidazole-1 acetamide (RO7-1051). The action of benznidazole is related to the nitroreduction of components of the parasite and the binding of metabolites to the nuclear DNA and k-DNA of *T. cruzi* and the lipids and proteins of the parasite.

Cruzipain = Also known as cruzain or GP57/51, is a member of the papain C1 family of cystein proteinases (CPs).

Chagas disease, or American trypanosomiasis = Is a potentially life-threatening illness caused by the protozoan parasite *Trypanosoma cruzi*.

Donor = A person in defined good health conditions who voluntarily donates blood or blood components, including plasma for fractionation.

Nifurtimox = (4 [(5- nitrofurfurylidene) amino]-3-methylthiomorpholine-1,1didioxide (Bayer 2502). The mechanism of action of nifurtimox involves the production of nitro-anion radicals, which, in the presence of oxygen, leave *T. cruzi* incapable of detoxifying free radicals.

Pyrethroids = Numerous synthetic organic compounds, mostly based on the chrysanthemate moiety of pyrethrum, having analogous neurotoxic modes of action causing rapid knockdown and insecticidal effects.

Triatomine bugs = The vectors of Chagas' disease parasites, live in cracks and crevices in the walls and ceilings of poorly built houses.

Vector Carrier of infection = Vector-borne pathogen cause disease; *e.g.Trypanosoma cruzi* causes Chagas disease, transmitted by vector kissing bugs.

Vector control = Is any method to limit or reduce the arthropods that transmit disease pathogens. The most common type of vector control is mosquito control through a number of core and supplementary strategies.

Zoonosis = Is any disease or infection that is naturally transmissible from vertebrate animals to humans.

REFERENCES

[1] OPS/OMS. 2006. [cited 7 July 2015]. Available at: http://www.bvsops.org.uy/pdf/chagas19.pdf. (OPS/HDM/CD/425-06)

[2] Organización Mundial de la Salud. 2009. [cited from July 2015]. Available at: http://www.paho.org/hq/index.php?option=com_docman&task=doc_view &gid=15377&Itemid=

[3] Organización Mundial de la Salud. 2010. [cited from July 2015]. Available at: http://apps.who.int/gb/ebwha/pdf_files/WHA63/A63_17-sp.pdf

[4] WHO. Sustaining the drive to overcome the global impact of neglected tropical diseases: second WHO report on neglected tropical diseases 2013. [cited from July 2015]. Available at: http://www.who.int/neglected_diseases/9789241564540/en/

[5] WHO. Chagas disease in LatinAmerica: an epidemiological update based on 2010 estimates Weekly epidemiological record 90(6): 33-44. [cited from July 2015]. Available at: http://www.who.int/wer/2015/wer9006.pdf

[6] Basile L, Jansà JM, Carlier Y, *et al.* Chagas disease in European countries: the challenge of a surveillance system. Euro Surveill 2011; 16(37): 19968.
[PMID: 21944556]

[7] Rassi A Jr, Rassi A, Marin-Neto JA. Chagas disease. Lancet 2010; 375(9723): 1388-402.
[http://dx.doi.org/10.1016/S0140-6736(10)60061-X] [PMID: 20399979]

[8] Chatelain E. Chagas disease drug discovery: toward a new era. J Biomol Screen 2015; 20(1): 22-35.
[http://dx.doi.org/10.1177/1087057114550585] [PMID: 25245987]

[9] Nunes MC, Dones W, Morillo CA, Encina JJ, Ribeiro AL. Chagas disease: an overview of clinical and epidemiological aspects. J Am Coll Cardiol 2013; 62(9): 767-76.
[http://dx.doi.org/10.1016/j.jacc.2013.05.046] [PMID: 23770163]

[10] Yadon ZE, Schmunis GA. Congenital Chagas disease: estimating the potential risk in the United States. Am J Trop Med Hyg 2009; 81(6): 927-33.
[http://dx.doi.org/10.4269/ajtmh.2009.09-0257] [PMID: 19996418]

[11] Investing to Overcome the Global Impact of Neglected Tropical Diseases Third WHO Report on Neglected Tropical Diseases . WHO/HTM/NTD/20151 2015. (cited:0+ 8 de julio 2015) Available at: http://apps.who.int/iris/.../1/9789241564861_eng.pdf

[12] WHO. Accelerating work To overcome the global impact of Neglected tropical diseases. A roadmap for implementation WHO/HTM/NTD/20121 2012. [cited July 2015]. Available at: http://www.who.int/neglected_diseases/en|ROADMAP|

[13] Chagas CR. Nova tripanozomiase humana. Estudos sobre a morfologia e o ciclo evolutivo do Schizotrypanum cruzi n.g., n.sp.,ajente etiolojico de nova entidade morbida do homem. Mem Inst Oswaldo Cruz 1909; 1(2): 159-218. [online]. [http://dx.doi.org/10.1590/S0074-02761909000200008]

[14] de Souza W. A short review on the morphology of *Trypanosoma cruzi*: from 1909 to 1999. Mem Inst Oswaldo Cruz 1999; 94 (Suppl. 1): 17-36. [http://dx.doi.org/10.1590/S0074-02761999000700003] [PMID: 10677689]

[15] Tyler KM, Engman DM. The life cycle of Trypanosoma cruzi revisited. Int J Parasitol 2001; 31(5-6): 472-81. [http://dx.doi.org/10.1016/S0020-7519(01)00153-9] [PMID: 11334932]

[16] UNAMF. de M., OPS, OMS. Manual para el Diagnostico de la Infección por *Trypanosoma cruzi*. OPS/OMS, México, p 45. 2006.

[17] Kowalska A, Kowalski P, Torres MA. Chagas disease-American trypanosomiasis. Polish Annals of Medicine 2011; 18: 156-67. [http://dx.doi.org/10.1016/S1230-8013(11)70035-2]

[18] Salazar-Schettino PM, Bucio MI, Cabrera M, Bautista J. First case of natural infection in pigs. Review of *Trypanosoma cruzi* reservoirs in Mexico. Mem Inst Oswaldo Cruz 1997; 92(4): 499-502. [http://dx.doi.org/10.1590/S0074-02761997000400010] [PMID: 9361743]

[19] Teixeira AR, Hecht MM, Guimaro MC, Sousa AO, Nitz N. Pathogenesis of chagas' disease: parasite persistence and autoimmunity. Clin Microbiol Rev 2011; 24(3): 592-630. [http://dx.doi.org/10.1128/CMR.00063-10] [PMID: 21734249]

[20] Frasch AC. Functional diversity in the trans-sialidase and mucin families in *Trypanosoma cruzi*. Parasitol Today (Regul Ed) 2000; 16(7): 282-6. [http://dx.doi.org/10.1016/S0169-4758(00)01698-7] [PMID: 10858646]

[21] de Souza W, de Carvalho TM, Barrias ES. Review on *Trypanosoma cruzi*: Host Cell Interaction. Int J Cell Biol 2010; 2010: 1-18. [http://dx.doi.org/10.1155/2010/295394] [PMID: 20811486]

[22] Osorio L, Ríos I, Gutiérrez B, González J. Virulence factors of *Trypanosoma cruzi*: who is who? Microbes Infect 2012; 14(15): 1390-402. [http://dx.doi.org/10.1016/j.micinf.2012.09.03] [PMID: 23006853]

[23] Yoshida N. Molecular basis of mammalian cell invasion by *Trypanosoma cruzi*. An Acad Bras Cienc 2006; 78(1): 87-111. [http://dx.doi.org/10.1590/S0001-37652006000100010] [PMID: 16532210]

[24] Maeda FY, Cortez C, Yoshida N. Cell signaling during *Trypanosoma cruzi* invasion. Front Immunol 2012; 3: 361. [http://dx.doi.org/10.3389/fimmu.2012.00361] [PMID: 23230440]

[25] Ortega-Barria E, Pereira ME. A novel *T. cruzi* heparin-binding protein promotes fibroblast adhesion and penetration of engineered bacteria and trypanosomes into mammalian cells. Cell 1991; 67(2): 411-21.
[http://dx.doi.org/10.1016/0092-8674(91)90192-2] [PMID: 1655283]

[26] Alvarez VE, Niemirowicz GT, Cazzulo JJ. The peptidases of Trypanosoma cruzi: Digestive enzymes, virulence factors, and mediators of autophagy and programmed cell death. Biochim Biophys Acta, Proteins Proteomics 2012; 1824: 195-206.

[27] Brisse S, Barnabé C, Bañuls AL, Sidibé I, Noël S, Tibayrenc M. A phylogenetic analysis of the *Trypanosoma cruzi* genome project CL Brener reference strain by multilocus enzyme electrophoresis and multiprimer random amplified polymorphic DNA fingerprinting. Mol Biochem Parasitol 1998; 92(2): 253-63.
[http://dx.doi.org/10.1016/S0166-6851(98)00005-X] [PMID: 9657330]

[28] Zingales B, Andrade SG, Briones MR, *et al.* A new consensus for *Trypanosoma cruzi* intraspecific nomenclature: second revision meeting recommends TcI to TcVI. Mem Inst Oswaldo Cruz 2009; 104(7): 1051-4.
[http://dx.doi.org/10.1590/S0074-02762009000700021] [PMID: 20027478]

[29] Burgos JM, Diez M, Vigliano C, *et al.* Molecular identification of *Trypanosoma cruzi* discrete typing units in end-stage chronic Chagas heart disease and reactivation after heart transplantation. Clin Infect Dis 2010; 51(5): 485-95.
[http://dx.doi.org/10.1086/655680] [PMID: 20645859]

[30] Schofield CJ, Galvão C. Classification, evolution, and species groups within the Triatominae. Acta Trop 2009; 110(2-3): 88-100.
[http://dx.doi.org/10.1016/j.actatropica.2009.01.010] [PMID: 19385053]

[31] WHO. Technical Report Series 905 Second report of the WHO Expert Committee Control of Chagas Disease [cited july 2015]. Available at: www.whqlibdoc.who.int/trs/WHO_TRS_905.pdf and CHAGAS-2002-WHO_TRS_905.pdf

[32] Lehane MJ. The Biology of Blood-Sucking in Insects. 2nd ed. Cambridge: University Press 2005; p. 321.
[http://dx.doi.org/10.1017/CBO9780511610493]

[33] Jurberg J, Galvão C. Biology, ecology, and systematics of Triatominae (Heteroptera, Reduviidae), vectors of Chagas disease, and implications for human health. Festschrift zum 70. Geburtstag von Ernst Heiss. Denisia 19, zugleich Katalogue der OÖ. Landesmuseen Neue Serie 2006; 50: 1095-116.

[34] Teixeira AR, Nascimento RJ, Sturm NR. Evolution and pathology in chagas disease--a review. Mem Inst Oswaldo Cruz 2006; 101(5): 463-91.
[http://dx.doi.org/10.1590/S0074-02762006000500001] [PMID: 17072450]

[35] Lent H, Wygodzinsky P. Revision of the Triatominae (Hemiptera, Reduviidae), and their significance as vectors of Chagas disease. Bull Am Mus Nat Hist 1979; 163: 123-520.

[36] Castillo D, Wolff M. Aspectos del comportamiento de los triatominos (Hemiptera: Reduviidae), vectores de la enfermedad de Chagas. Biomedica 2000; 20: 59-64.
[http://dx.doi.org/10.7705/biomedica.v20i1.1048]

[37] Galvão C, Carcavallo R, Da Silva Rocha D, Jurberg J. A checklist of the current valid species of the subfamily Triatominae Jeannel, 1919 (Hemiptera, Reduviidae) and their geographical distribution, with nomenclatural and taxonomic notes. Zootaxa 2003; 202: 1-36.

[38] Salazar-Schettino PM, Rojas G, Cabrera M, *et al.* A revision of thirteen species of Triatominae (Hemiptera: Reduviidae) vectors of Chagas disease in Mexico. Journal of the Selva Andina Research Society 2010; 1: 57-80.

[39] OPS/OMS. Información general: Enfermedad de Chagas, abril 2014 2014. [cited July 2015]. Available at: http://www.paho.org/hq/index.php?option=com_content&view=article&id=5856&Itemid=&lang=es

[40] Schaub GA, Meiser CK, Balczun C. Interactions of *Trypanosoma cruzi* and Triatomines. Progress in Parasitology 2011; 2: 155-78.

[41] Kollien AH, Schmidt J, Schaub GA. Modes of association of *Trypanosoma cruzi* with the intestinal tract of the vector *Triatoma infestans.* Acta Trop 1998; 70(2): 127-41. [http://dx.doi.org/10.1016/S0001-706X(97)00117-4] [PMID: 9698259]

[42] Alves CR, Albuquerque-Cunha JM, Mello CB, *et al. Trypanosoma cruzi*: attachment to perimicrovillar membrane glycoproteins of *Rhodnius prolixus.* Exp Parasitol 2007; 116(1): 44-52. [http://dx.doi.org/10.1016/j.exppara.2006.11.012] [PMID: 17250827]

[43] Albuquerque-Cunha JM, Gonzalez MS, Garcia ES, *et al.* Cytochemical characterization of microvillar and perimicrovillar membranes in the posterior midgut epithelium of *Rhodnius prolixus.* Arthropod Struct Dev 2009; 38(1): 31-44. [http://dx.doi.org/10.1016/j.asd.2008.06.001] [PMID: 18602023]

[44] OMS/TDR. Reporte sobre la enfermedad de Chagas Grupo de trabajo científico 17 a 20 de abril de 2005 Actualizado en julio de 2007. Buenos Aires Argentina. [cited July 2015]. Available at: http://whqlibdoc.who.int/hq/2007/TDR_SWG_09_spa.pdf

[45] Moncayo A. Progress towards interruption of transmission of Chagas disease. Mem Inst Oswaldo Cruz 1999; 94 (Suppl. 1): 401-4. [http://dx.doi.org/10.1590/S0074-02761999000700079] [PMID: 10677765]

[46] Cardoni R, Antúnez M, Abrami A. Respuesta TH1 en la infección experimental con Trypanosoma cruzi. Medicina (Buenos Aires) 1999; 59 (Suppl II): 84-90.

[47] Kierszenbaum F. Views on the autoimmunity hypothesis for Chagas disease pathogenesis. FEMS Immunol Med Microbiol 2003; 37(1): 1-11. [http://dx.doi.org/10.1016/S0928-8244(03)00097-X] [PMID: 12770754]

[48] Gutiérrez FR, Guedes PM, Gazzinelli RT, Silva JS. The role of parasite persistence in pathogenesis of Chagas heart disease. Parasite Immunol 2009; 31(11): 673-85. [http://dx.doi.org/10.1111/j.1365-3024.2009.01108.x] [PMID: 19825107]

[49] Araujo-Jorge TC, Waghabi MC, Soeiro MN, Keramidas M, Bailly S, Feige JJ. Pivotal role for TGF-β in infectious heart disease: the case of *Trypanosoma cruzi* infection and its consequent chagasic cardiomyopathy. Cytokine Growth Factor Rev 2008; 19: 405-13.

[50] Köberle F. Chagas' disease and Chagas' syndromes: the pathology of American trypanosomiasis. Adv Parasitol 1968; 6: 63-116.

[http://dx.doi.org/10.1016/S0065-308X(08)60472-8] [PMID: 4239747]

[51] Marín-Neto JA, Cunha-Neto E, Maciel BC, Simões MV. Pathogenesis of chronic Chagas heart disease. Circulation 2007; 115(9): 1109-23. [http://dx.doi.org/10.1161/CIRCULATIONAHA.106.624296] [PMID: 17339569]

[52] Marin-Neto JA, Rassi A Jr. Actualización sobre la cardiopatía de la enfermedad de Chagas en el primer centenario de su descubrimiento. Rev Esp Cardiol 2009; 62: 1211-6. [http://dx.doi.org/10.1016/S0300-8932(09)73071-4] [PMID: 19889330]

[53] Herrera RN, Díaz E, Pérez R, *et al.* Estado protrombótico en estadios tempranos de la enfermedad de Chagas crónica. Rev Esp Cardiol 2003; 56(4): 377-82. [http://dx.doi.org/10.1016/S0300-8932(03)76881-X] [PMID: 12689572]

[54] Torres CM. Sobre a anatomia patológica da doença de Chagas. Mem Inst Oswaldo Cruz 1941; 36: 391-404. [http://dx.doi.org/10.1590/S0074-02761941000300015]

[55] Tafuri WL. Patogenia da doença de Chagas. Rev Inst Med Trop Sao Paulo 1987; 29(4): 194-9. [http://dx.doi.org/10.1590/S0036-46651987000400002] [PMID: 3130653]

[56] Cunha-Neto E, Bilate AM, Hyland KV, Fonseca SG, Kalil J, Engman DM. Induction of cardiac autoimmunity in Chagas heart disease: a case for molecular mimicry. Autoimmunity 2006; 39: 41-5. [http://dx.doi.org/10.1080/08916930500485002]

[57] Borda ES, Sterin-Borda L. Antiadrenergic and muscarinic receptor antibodies in Chagas' cardiomyopathy. Int J Cardiol 1996; 54(2): 149-56. [http://dx.doi.org/10.1016/0167-5273(96)02592-2] [PMID: 8803679]

[58] Guerreiro C, Machado A. Da reação de Bordet et Gengou na molestia de Carlos Chagas como elemento diagnostico. Bras Med 1913; 27(23): 225-6.

[59] Boyden SV. The adsorption of proteins on erythrocytes treated with tannic acid and subsequent hemagglutination by antiprotein sera. J Exp Med 1951; 93(2): 107-20. [http://dx.doi.org/10.1084/jem.93.2.107] [PMID: 14803635]

[60] Camargo ME. Fluorescent antibody test for the serodiagnosis of American trypanosomiasis. Technical modification employing preserved culture forms of Trypanosoma cruzi in a slide test. Rev Inst Med Trop Sao Paulo 1966; 8(5): 227-35. [PMID: 4967348]

[61] Voller A, Draper C, Bidwell DE, Bartlett A. Microplate enzyme-linked immunosorbent assay for chagas' disease. Lancet 1975; 1(7904): 426-8. [http://dx.doi.org/10.1016/S0140-6736(75)91492-0] [PMID: 48613]

[62] Viotti RJ, Vigliano C, Laucella C, *et al.* Value of echocardiogram for diagnosis and prognosis of chronic chagasic miocarditis without heart failure. 2004 90: 655-60.

[63] Apt W, Zulantay I. Estado actual en el tratamiento de la enfermedad de Chagas. Rev Med Chil 2011; 139(2): 247-57. [http://dx.doi.org/10.4067/S0034-98872011000200016] [PMID: 21773664]

[64] Murcia L, Carrilero B, Albajar Viñas P, Segovia M. Nifurtimox chemotherapy: collateral effects in treated *Trypanosoma cruzi* infected patients. Rev Esp Quimioter 2012; 25(1): 74-5.

[PMID: 22488545]

[65] [cited 8th July 2015]. Available at: http://www.dndi.org/diseases-projects/diseases/chagas.html.

[66] WHO monographs on selected medicinal plants Vol. 4 [homepage on the internet]. . Geneva 2009. [cited: 23rd July 2015]. Available at: http://apps.who.int/medicinedocs/es/m/abstract/Js16713e/

[67] Berger I, Barrientos AC, Cáceres A, *et al.* Plants used in Guatemala for the treatment of protozoal infections: II. Activity of extracts and fractions of five Guatemalan plants against Trypanosoma cruzi. J Ethnopharmacol 1998; 62(2): 107-15. [http://dx.doi.org/10.1016/S0378-8741(98)00011-7] [PMID: 9741882]

[68] Muelas-Serrano S, Nogal JJ, Martínez-Díaz RA, Escario JA, Martínez-Fernández AR, Gómez-Barrio A. *In vitro* screening of american plant extracts on *Trypanosoma cruzi* and *trichomonas vaginalis.* J Ethnopharmacol 2000; 71(1-2): 101-7. [http://dx.doi.org/10.1016/S0378-8741(99)00185-3] [PMID: 10904152]

[69] Pizzolatti MG, Koga AH, Grisard EC, Steindel M. Trypanocidal activity of extracts from Brazilian Atlantic Rain Forest plant species. Phytomedicine 2003; 10(5): 422-6. [http://dx.doi.org/10.1078/0944-7113-00252] [PMID: 12834008]

[70] Paveto C, Güida MC, Esteva MI, *et al.* Anti-*Trypanosoma cruzi* activity of green tea (*Camellia sinensis*) catechins. Antimicrob Agents Chemother 2004; 48(1): 69-74. [http://dx.doi.org/10.1128/AAC.48.1.69-74.2004] [PMID: 14693520]

[71] Ruiz PG, Garavito G, Acebey L, *et al.* Actividad Leishmanicida y Tripanocida de algunas plantas reportadas como medicinales en Colombia BIOFARBO 2004.

[72] Schinor EC, Salvador MJ, Ito IY, de Albuquerque S, Dias DA. Trypanocidal and antimicrobial activities of *Moquinia kingii.* Phytomedicine 2004; 11(2-3): 224-9. [http://dx.doi.org/10.1078/0944-7113-00342] [PMID: 15070176]

[73] Tenorio JL, Hernández JE, Vallejo A, Dairo J. Actividad tripanomicida en el Trypanosoma cruzi del extracto etanólico de las semillas de la Xylopia aromatica. Rev Cubana Farm 2006; 40(3): 224-9. [serial on the Internet]. [cited July 29, 2015]. Available at: http://scielo.sld.cu/scielo.php?script=sci_arttext&pid=S0034-75152006000300008&lng=en

[74] Santoro GF, Cardoso MG, Guimarães LG, Freire JM, Soares MJ. Anti-proliferative effect of the essential oil of *Cymbopogon citratus* (DC) Stapf (lemongrass) on intracellular amastigotes, bloodstream trypomastigotes and culture epimastigotes of *Trypanosoma cruzi* (Protozoa: Kinetoplastida). Parasitology 2007; 134(Pt 11): 1649-56. [http://dx.doi.org/10.1017/S0031182007002958] [PMID: 17686189]

[75] Santoro GF, das Graças Cardoso M, Guimarães LG, Salgado AP, Menna-Barreto RF, Soares MJ. Effect of oregano (*Origanum vulgare* L.) and thyme (*Thymus vulgaris* L.) essential oils on *Trypanosoma cruzi* (Protozoa: Kinetoplastida) growth and ultrastructure. Parasitol Res 2007; 100(4): 783-90. [http://dx.doi.org/10.1007/s00436-006-0326-5] [PMID: 17024354]

[76] Santoro GF, Cardoso MG, Guimarães LG, Mendonça LZ, Soares MJ. *Trypanosoma cruzi*: activity of essential oils from *Achillea millefolium* L., *Syzygium aromaticum* L. and *Ocimum basilicum* L. on epimastigotes and trypomastigotes. Exp Parasitol 2007; 116(3): 283-90.

[http://dx.doi.org/10.1016/j.exppara.2007.01.018] [PMID: 17349626]

[77] Cardoso J, Soares MJ. *In vitro* effects of citral on trypanosoma cruzi metacyclogenesis. Mem Inst Oswaldo Cruz 2010; 105(8): 1026-32.
[http://dx.doi.org/10.1590/S0074-02762010000800012] [PMID: 21225200]

[78] Rojas J, Solís H, Palacios O. Evaluación *in vitro* de la actividad anti *Trypanosoma cruzi* de aceites esenciales de diez plantas medicinales. An Fac Med 2010; 71: 161-5.

[79] Valencia L, Muñoz DL, Robledo SM, *et al.* Actividad tripanocida y citotóxica de extractos de plantas colombianas. Biomedica 2011; 31(4): 552-9.
[http://dx.doi.org/10.7705/biomedica.v31i4.426] [PMID: 22674366]

[80] Grecco SdosS, Reimão JQ, Tempone AG, *et al. In vitro* antileishmanial and antitrypanosomal activities of flavanones from *Baccharis retusa* DC. (Asteraceae). Exp Parasitol 2012; 130(2): 141-5.
[http://dx.doi.org/10.1016/j.exppara.2011.11.002] [PMID: 22143090]

[81] Rojas J, Ronceros S, Palacios O, Sevilla C. Efecto anti-Trypanosoma cruzi del aceite esencial de *Cymbopogon citrates* (DC) Stapf (hierba luisa) en ratones Balb/c. An Fac Med 2012; 73: 7-12.

[82] Borges AR, Aires JR, Higino TM, *et al.* Trypanocidal and cytotoxic activities of essential oils from medicinal plants of Northeast of Brazil. Exp Parasitol 2012; 132(2): 123-8.
[http://dx.doi.org/10.1016/j.exppara.2012.06.003] [PMID: 22771867]

[83] Hamuy R, Acosta N, López E, Ferreira ME, Vera de Bilbao N. Determinación de la sensibilidad *in vitro* de diferentes cepas de Trypanosoma cruzi al benznidazole y al extracto de hoja de la planta *Zanthoxylum chiloperone.* Mem Inst Investig Cienc Salud 2013; 11: 16-25.

[84] Veiga-Santos P, Desoti VC, Miranda N, *et al.* The natural compounds piperovatine and piperlonguminine induce autophagic cell death on *Trypanosoma cruzi.* Acta Trop 2013; 125(3): 349-56.
[http://dx.doi.org/10.1016/j.actatropica.2012.11.014] [PMID: 23228524]

[85] da Silva Ferreira D, Rodrigues V, Marçal MG, *et al.* Natural products and Chagas' disease: the action of triterpenes acids isolated from *Miconia* species. Universitas Scientiarum 2013; 18: 243-56.
[http://dx.doi.org/10.11144/Javeriana.SC18-2.npcd]

[86] Bou DD, Tempone AG, Pinto ÉG, Lago JH, Sartorelli P. Antiparasitic activity and effect of casearins isolated from *Casearia sylvestris* on Leishmania and *Trypanosoma cruzi* plasma membrane. Phytomedicine 2014; 21(5): 676-81.
[http://dx.doi.org/10.1016/j.phymed.2014.01.004] [PMID: 24560122]

[87] Molina-Garza ZJ, Bazaldúa-Rodríguez AF, Quintanilla-Licea R, Galaviz-Silva L. Anti-*Trypanosoma cruzi* activity of 10 medicinal plants used in northeast Mexico. Acta Trop 2014; 136: 14-8.
[http://dx.doi.org/10.1016/j.actatropica.2014.04.006] [PMID: 24742906]

[88] Azeredo CM, Santos T, Lameiro de Noronha Sales Maia BH, Soares MJ. *In vitro* biological evaluation of eight different essential oils against Trypanosoma cruzi, with emphasis on Cinnamomum verum essential oil. BMC Complementary and Alternative 2015. (cited 24 de junio 2015). Available at: http://www.biomedcentral.com/1472-6882/14/309

[89] Silva CV, Bomfim FC, Dos Santos MA, *et al.* Estudo fitoquímico e avaliação *in vitro* da atividade anti-*Trypanosoma cruzi* cepa Y de *Pilocarpus spicatus St. Hil. (Rutaceae).* Rev Bras Pl Med Campinas

2014; 16: 812-8.
[http://dx.doi.org/10.1590/1983-084X/11_112]

[90] Martínez R, Escribano A, Burillo J, *et al.* Trypanocidal, trichomonacidal and cytotoxic components of cultivated Artemisia absinthium Linnaeus (Asteraceae) essential oil. Mem Inst Oswaldo Cruz 2015; 1-7. Available at: http://memorias.ioc.fiocruz.br.
[http://dx.doi.org/10.1590/0074- 02760140129]

[91] Izumi E, Ueda-Nakamura T, Dias Filho BP, Veiga Júnior VF, Nakamura CV. Natural products and Chagas' disease: a review of plant compounds studied for activity against *Trypanosoma cruzi.* Nat Prod Rep 2011; 28(4): 809-23.
[http://dx.doi.org/10.1039/c0np00069h] [PMID: 21290079]

[92] McCulley SF, Setzer WN. An *in-silico* investigation of anti-Chagas phytochemicals. Curr Clin Pharmacol 2014; 9(3): 205-57.
[http://dx.doi.org/10.2174/157488470903140806114147] [PMID: 23173969]

[93] Centers for Disease Control and Prevention. Chagas Disease [homepage on the internet] Atlanta, GA [cited 14th July 2015]. Available at: http://www.cdc.gov/parasites/chagas/biology.html

CHAPTER 4

Malaria, Generalities and New Treatments

Luz Eugenia Alcántara-Quintana[1,*], Mónica Salas-Rojas[2] and Emmanuelle Alvarado-Alvarez[3]

[1] *Potosino Institute for Scientific Research, Road to San José Dam 4th 2055. AP. 78216, San Luis Potosi, Mexico*

[2] *National Medical Center, XXI Century, Mexican Social Security Institute. Doctores 330, Cuauhtemoc, AP. 06725, Mexico City, Mexico*

[3] *Centre for Science and Technology Studies 14, Luis Enrique Erro, National Polytechnic Institute, Michoacana, Venustiano Carranza, AP. 15240, Mexico City, Mexico*

Abstract: Malaria is still a grave public health problem in tropical areas of the world. The greater genetic diversity of *Plasmodium vivax* at geographic sites with less control over infection reveals the importance of genetic studies of these parasites. *Plasmodium vivax* is the main cause of human malaria in Asia and Latin America but is absent from most of central Africa due to the near fixation of a mutation that inhibits the expression of its receptor, the Duffy antigen, on human erythrocytes. The search for vaccine development remains an issue of global concern.

Keywords: Dufy antigen, Malaria, New Treatments, *Plasmodium vivax*, Quinine, Vaccines.

MALARIA GENERALITIES

Malaria is an acute or chronic tropical disease caused by protozoans of the genus *Plasmodium*. This protozoan occurs in red blood cells. The hosts of *Plasmodium* are humans and other mammals as well as reptiles and birds. Malaria in humans is caused by five species of *Plasmodium*: *Plasmodium falciparum*, occurring mainly

* **Corresponding author Alcántara-Quintana LE:** Molecular Biology, Potosino Institute for Scientific Research, Road to San José Dam 4th 2055. AP. 78216, San Luis Potosi, Mexico; Tel: 52 (444) 834 20 00 ; E-mail: luz.alcantara@ipicyt.edu.mx

Norma Rivera (Ed.)

in countries with a tropical climate, in particular in Sub-Saharan Africa (south and center of the continent); *Plasmodium vivax*, having the broadest range of occurrence (from the tropical to the moderate zone); *Plasmodium malariae*, occurring sporadically in countries with a subtropical and tropical climate; *Plasmodium ovale*, occurring in the west of Africa, the Philippines, east of Indonesia and in Papua New Guinea; and *Plasmodium knowlesi*, occurring in south-east Asia, Singapore, Malaysia and Thailand. Among the five species, the most dangerous is *Plasmodium falciparum* .

In the malarian transmission approximately 30–40 species of mosquitoes of the genus *Anopheles* fulfill the significant role of vectors. The mosquitoes responsible for spreading the disease breed in various bodies of water; they like puddles and also rice fields. The number of mosquitoes depends on a large extent on the rainfall intensity, temperature and humidity. The most suitable conditions for mosquito development and malaria transmission are the air temperature of 17–33 °C and the mean relative humidity above 60%. Most blood- sucking mosquitoes are crepuscular feeders [1].

Plasmodium Life Cycle

The Life Cycle is almost the same for all the species that infect humans (Fig. **1**).

In humans, the parasites grow and multiply first in the liver cells and then in the blood red cells. In the blood, successive broods of parasites grow inside the red cells and destroy them, releasing daughter parasites ("merozoites") that continue the cycle by invading other red cells [2 - 5].

The blood stage parasites are those that cause the symptoms of malaria. When certain forms of blood stage parasites ("gametocytes") are picked up by a female *Anopheles* mosquito during a blood meal, they start another, different cycle of growth and multiplication in the mosquito [2 - 5].

After 10-18 days, the parasites are found (as "sporozoites") in the mosquito's salivary glands. When the *Anopheles* mosquito takes a blood meal on another human, the sporozoites are injected with the mosquito's saliva and start another human infection when they parasitize the liver cells [6 - 9].

Thus the mosquito carries the disease from one human to another (acting as a "vector"). Differently from the human host, the mosquito vector does not suffer from the presence of the parasites [6 - 9].

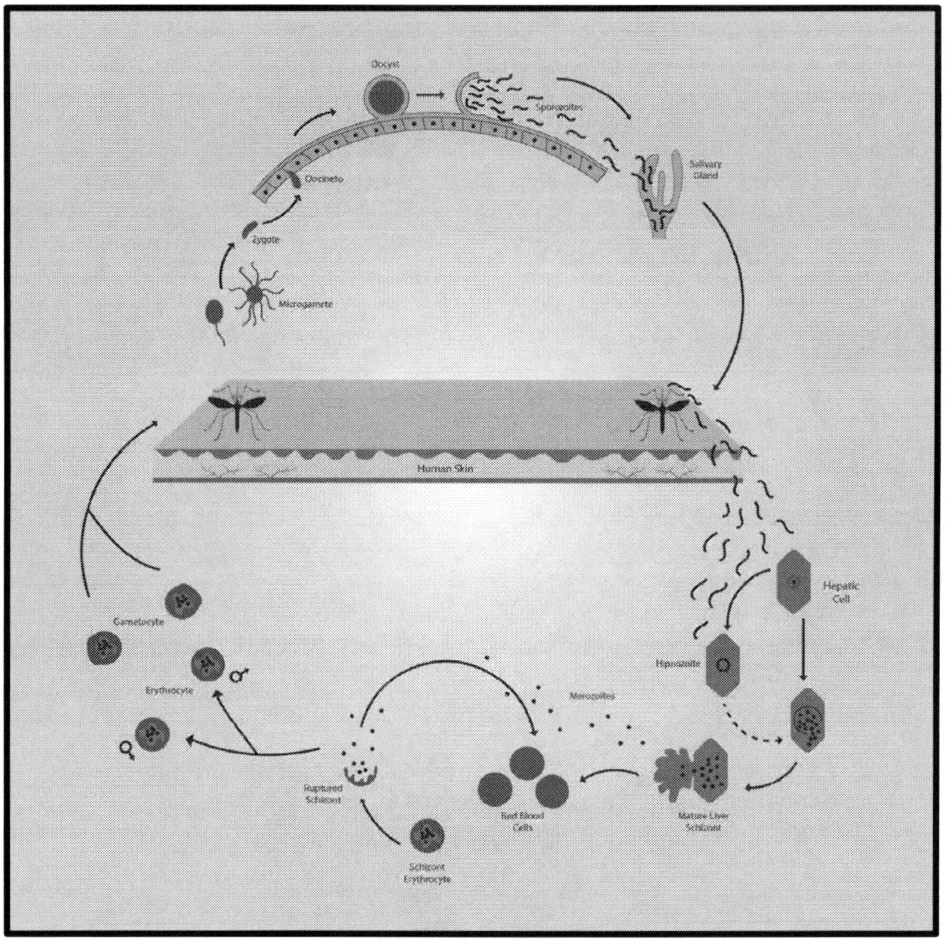

Fig. (1). Life cycle of the malaria parasite. (Modified by Alcántara-Quintana L, of the one of a series 'Malaria: Parasite Biology Tutorial', www.wellcome.ac.uk) [2 - 5].

NEW TREATMENTS

Quinine was the first natural antimalarial agent, this compound is an alkaloyd extracted from the bark of the cinchona tree (*Cinchona calisaya*) [10]. The first records from 1600's mention that the bark was used to make infusions and it was referred to as the "Jesuits' bark", "cardinal's bark", or 'sacred bark'; in 1820 it was first isolated by Pierre Joseph Pelletier and Joseph Caventou remaining as the main treatment [11]. In the 1890's, Paul Erlich used methylene blue to treat malaria patients by its selective capacity to be absorbed by the parasites; also, in the 1920's, Erlich synthesized quinine analogues, obtaining various compounds some of which resulted too toxic to be used [10]. Chloroquine synthesis was achieved during the World War II, this drug is used nowadays due to its high efficiency despite the fact that there are some resistant *P. falciparum* and *P. vivax* to it; then hydroxychloroquine was discovered, which turned out to be a less toxic drug and therefore a good treatment alternative [10].

Currently arthemisinin-based therapies are used, this compound was discovered in the 70's, but its use goes back to Traditional Chinese Medicine which employs the Qing Hao (*Artemisia annua*) for fever treatment [12 - 18]. The current recommendation is to use this compound combined with another (ACT, arthemisinin-based combination therapy), because in Asia some resistance was found when used alone [19]. There are also non-arthemisinin-based combination therapies [19], if resistance is present or drugs are not available.

Quinine

It's a basic alkaloid that exists in various preparations, including the hydrochloride, dihydrochloride, sulfate, bisulfate and gluconate salts [7]. This drug has a rapid schizonticidal action against intra-erithrocytic malaria parasites due to an hemzoin biocrystallization inhibitory activity. It is also gametocytocidal for *Plasmodium vivax* and *P. malariae* [11, 19]. It is used both oral and parentally, it is highly protein bound to alpha-1 acid glycoprotein, reaching peak concentrations within 1 to 3 hours and a half -life of 11 to 18 hours [11]. One reason why its use has decreased is because some drugs with less side effects or milder adverse reactions were developed. Some of these mild side effects include cinchonism, slight impairment of hearing, headache, nausea, hypoglycemia and the more severe include vertigo, vomiting, abdominal pain, diarrhea, marked auditory loss and visual symptoms. Less frequent include skin eruptions, asthma, thrombocytopaenia, hepatic injury and psychosis [11].

The Centers for Disease Control and Prevention (CDC) recommended treatment for uncomplicated malaria quinine sulfate plus either Doxycycline or Tetracycline or Clindamycin just in case of Chloroquine resistance. Treatment for infections acquired in Southeast Asia should continue for 7 days and for those acquired in Africa or South America should continue for 3 days [20]. Docycycline and Tetracycline are not indicated for use in children less than 8 years old; the use of Quinin plus Clindamycine is for pregnant women with a chloroquine-resistant infection [20]. A treatment table is available at http://www.cdc.gov./malaria/resources/pdf/treatmenttable.pdf.

Furthermore, the World Health Organization (WHO) for uncomplicated malaria recommends using quinine plus clincamycine for 7 days for pregnant women in their first trimester infected with chloroquine-resistant strains, and quinine can even be used alone if there is no clindamycin available [21].

In the same treatment guidelines states the recommendation of quinine plus either tetracycline or doxycycline or clindamycin for recurrences occurring beyond 28 days of the first treatment [21].

In addition to side reactions produced by quinine, the development of more potent and less toxic drugs (and therefore with simpler or shorter application schemes) led to recommend its use only in special cases and/or lack of other drugs, since the latter have greater success in treatment compliance [11, 20, 21]. Chemical structure of quinine is depicted in Fig. (**2**).

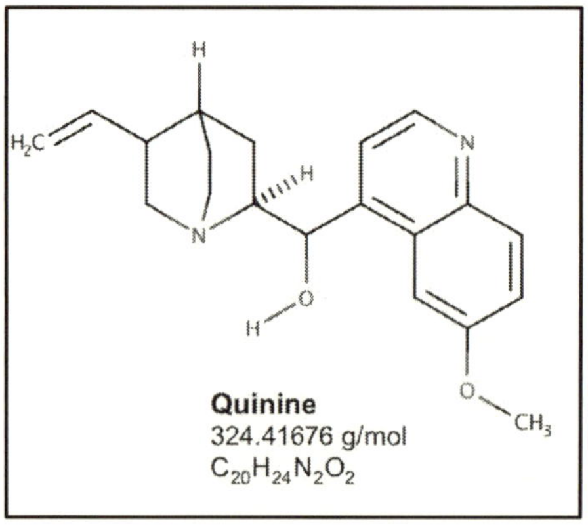

Fig. (2). 2D-Structures of quininine, malarial drug used for treatment. Self-constructed based on NCBI Pubchem with computer program, Chem Axon [13 - 14].

Chloroquine

Chloroquine (Fig. **3**) is one of the main drugs in the fight against malaria, but resistance cases to it have established the difference to treat patients. This drug belongs to the aminoquinoline group. In some countries, chloroquine analogues are used as a preventive treatment. Chloroquine analogues are water soluble and absorbed in the gastrointestinal tract, with peak plasma concentration of 4 to 12 hours and a half-life of 40 to 50 days [10]. This drugs can bound to plasma proteins, mainly albumin and α-acid glycoprotein. Excretion is quite slow and mostly excreted by urine, but also can be found in saliva and sweat [10]. Some of the side effects include retinopathy, cardiomyopathy, neuromyopathy and myopathy; although these are rare and occur mainly when the drug is administered in high doses and very rapidly by parental routes [10]. Chloroquine acts only on erythrocytic stages of *P. falciparum* lowering blood levels of the parasite without affecting the other stages [22].

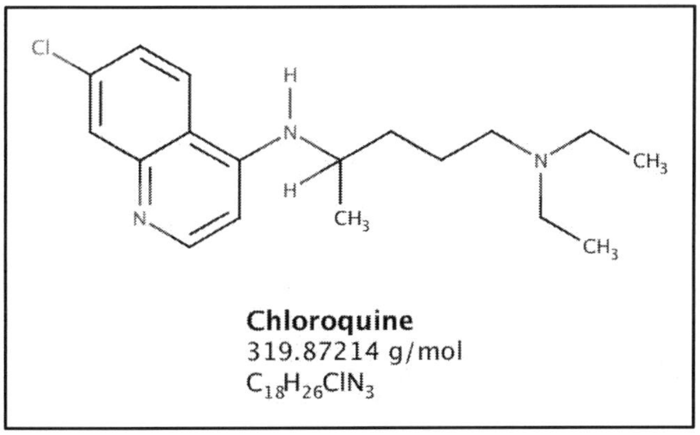

Fig. (3). 2D-Structures of chloroquine, malarial drug used for treatment. Self-constructed based on NCBI Pubchem with computer program, Chem Axon [14, 15].

In the CDC guidelines for treatment of patients with uncomplicated malaria infected with chloroquine-sensitive strains (Central America, Haiti, the Dominican Republic, and most of the Middle East) administration of oral chloroquine to a total dose of 1500 mg in 48 hours; another option is to use hydroxychloroquine up to a total dose of 1550 mg in 48 hours [20]. For further details refer to the treatment table cited previously on the text.

The use of chloroquine or hydroxychloroquine is also recommended for infections of *P. vivax* and *P. ovale* acquired in Asia, except for those acquired in Papua New Guinea and Indonesia, because in those areas chloroquine-resistant strains occur [20]. Pregnant patients with uncomplicated malaria infected with chloroquine-sensitive strains should be treated as mentioned above, even in cases of pregnant patients with *P. vivax* or *P. ovale* infections should be maintained on chloroquine prophylaxis for the duration of their pregnancy (300 mg orally once per week) [20].

Furthermore, the WHO, instead of chloroquine uses artemisinin-based combination therapy (ACT) [21]. For uncomplicated malaria treatment as will be seen later on this chapter. These guidelines mention chloroquine as treatment of uncomplicated malaria caused by *P. vivax, P. malariae* and *P. knowlesi* [21].

Artemisinin

Artemisinin (Fig. **4**) is a sesquiterpene lactone bearing a peroxy group, the active metabolite of artemisinin is dihydroartemisinin (DHA). The clinical treatment includes DHA, artemether, artesunate and arteether [23]. The peroxide bridge is the active group of artemisinin, which breaks down by reacting with heme or free iron. This bridge allows the artemisinin molecule to react with the free radicals that are increased in infected cells, resulting in an enhance of drug permissibility in those cells and less reaction in uninfected cells and therefore produces fewer side reactions [18 - 23].

CDC guidelines for treatment of malaria recommend among its two first treatments for uncomplicated malaria the administration of artemether plus lumefantrine orally for 3 days only if *Plasmodium* species is chloroquine-resistant, except pregnant patients and children less than 8 years old [20].

In a contrasting way, WHO, in its guidelines for the treatment of uncomplicated malaria, base their scheme in ACT (Artemisinin-based Combination Therapy) with regimens that provide a 3 days treatment with an artemisinin derivative, except pregnant women in their first trimester [21]. To treat severe malaria cases applying intravenous or intramuscular artesunate for at least 24 hours is recommended, followed by oral ACT when tolerated [21]. Thus, artemisinin derivatives are still recommended by WHO as antimalarials. However, it has been reported that in some patients, artesunate administration can develop delayed haemolysis [24].

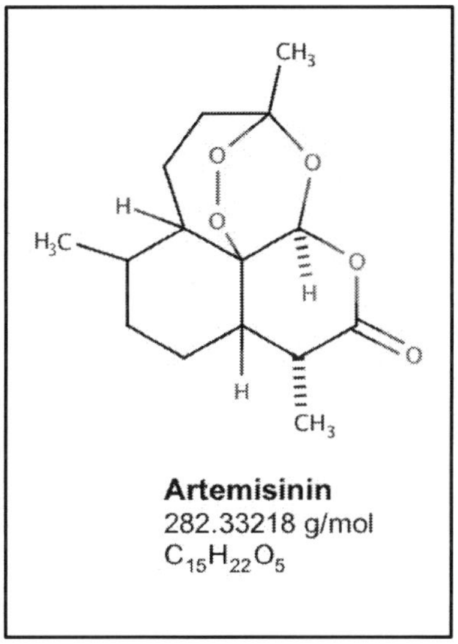

Fig. (4). 2D-Structures of artemisinin, malarial drug used for treatment. Self-constructed based on NCBI Pubchem with computer program, Chem Axon [14 - 16].

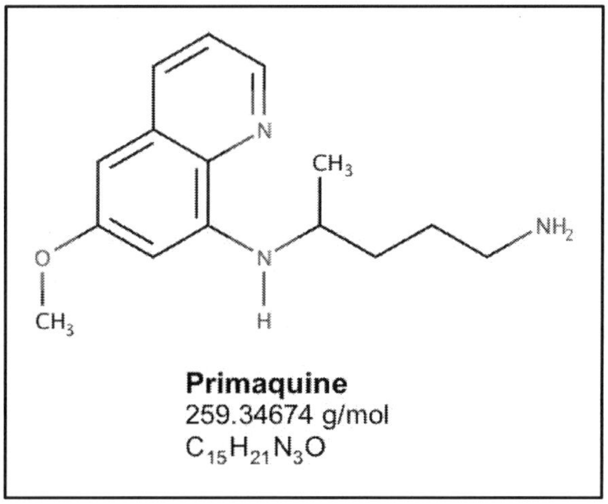

Fig. (5). 2D-Structures of primaquine, malarial drug used for treatment. Self-constructed based on NCBI Pubchem with computer program, Chem Axon [14 - 17].

Primaquine

Primaquine (Fig. **5**) is part of some of the previous referred treatments and it is administered preventing relapse due to the release of hyponozoites that may remain dormant in the liver [20, 21]. However, one special condition to consider (besides pregnant and nursing women, children under 8 years old or less than 5 Kg/weight) is the G6PD (Glucose-6-Phosphate Dehydrogenase) deficiency status of patients since primaquine treatment will experience haemolysis but the severity of haemolysis may vary depending on the dose of primaquine and the variant of the G6PD enzyme [21].

Resistance

Resistance to antimalarial drugs is of great interest; various approaches have been made to this topic, from compliance of treatment, epidemiological and genetic studies to determine drug susceptibility, strain mobility and the best management and/or control to prevent treatment abandonment.

A review study about treatment compliance in malaria patients, emphasizes that the rapid and proper diagnosis, drug prescription and the right dose, drugs' availability in health institutions and the proper intake (dose and timing) by patients is important to prevent relapse episodes and treatment resistant parasite selection [25].

Chloroquine is one of the most widely used drugs against malaria since 1950's, and is the safest treatment for pregnant women and 8 years old children [22]. However, 10 years after its first use, some chloroquine-resistant *Plasmodium falciparum* infection cases were documented in Southeast Asia and South America; by the 1980's this has spread to almost all countries with *P. falciparum* [11]. Epidemiological studies showed that chloroquine-resistance was originated in 6 different foci distributed among Africa, Southeast Asia and Latin America [26].

Up to date only one case of chlorquine-resistance in *P. malariae* has been reported in Indonesia, confirmed by PCR amplification, where the adequate management and absorption of drug was ensured [27].

To understand the molecule responsible for conferring resistance to *Plasmodium* strains two main targets have been described: PfCRT (*Plasmodium falciparum* Chloroquine-Resistance Transporter) and PfMDR (*Plasmodium falciparum* Multi-drug Resistance), both of which have been identified as the primary determinant of chloroquine and other drugs resistance [26, 28]. Both genes encode transport proteins, which are involved in the availability and metabolism of drug administration [26]. However, the presence of a mutation or allele within different genes is not enough to confer total drug resistance: *i.e.* many cases require more than one mutation and over one different gene for the strain to be resistant [26, 28]. This regulation led to the use of the term 'Tolerance to Chloroquine', that is, parasite susceptibility to chloroquine decreases and relapse events occur in chloroquine concentrations that would normally be lethal to the parasite [28].

The most common mutation associated with resistance to chloroquine is K76T in PfCRT protein, although other mutations have also been found in drug resistant strains [28 - 30]. The proposed mechanisms of action to confer resistance are that the mutated form of PfCRT reduces chloroquine accumulation in digestive vacuoles, while Pfmdrl (multi-drug resistance 1 gene) causes this drug to be sequestered in vacuolar compartments avoiding its action [30]. Both PfCRT and Pfmdr1 mechanisms is what gives patterns of resistance.

As it was mentioned before, ACT is the base treatment for malaria recommended by WHO. This drug is fast acting and very effective; however, in 2009 it was reported, on the border of Cambodia with Thailand, a decrease in rapid parasite clearance in patients [31]. Although a molecular marker that confers this resistance has not yet been found, it was detected a simple change in the gene that encodes a Kelch protein called K13 [32]. This protein is not unique to the parasite and belongs to a family of proteins with diverse functions. Besides, other genome changes in its genome have also been detected, so that their relevance is still being studied [32].

For other anti-malarial drugs used (not as massive as chloroquine or ACT) as treatment, some cases of resistance have been reported; *i.e.* resistance to atovaquone is associated to a mutation (Y268C or Y268S) of cytochrome b gene, however this is rare [30]. For sulfadoxine-pyrimethamine four mutations have been reported in the gene dihydrofolate reductase (DHFR), N51I/C59R/S108N/164L; however, the presence of the third one is enough to confer resistance to pyrimethamine [30]. Although this drug resistance to registered treatments, is the only recommended for pregnant women [21, 30].

One of the drugs for which there are no yet reported cases of resistance is primaquine [30].

The massive use of drugs and treatments based only on one of them is one of the causes that have led to the rising of resistant strains, so the current WHO recommendation to implement ACT as a base treatment is to avoid its extension since the resistance is registered.

CONCLUSION

Malaria is one of the most important parasitic diseases in tropical and subtropical areas of the world, in 2015 approximately 214 million cases were reported and due to prevention and control campaigns recorded a decrease in the mortality rate over 60% compared with data for the year 2000 [29]. Although the first reports of treatments, dating from the 17th century (with the use of infusions of the bark of the cinchona tree) to date, are still developing new drugs that are more effective, especially with the *Plasmodium* strains resistant to existing ones.

Examples are drugs currently used for treatment; is first the case of chloroquine, which use with the emergence of strains resistant to quinine was promoted; and artemisinin, which is now used in combination with another drug (to avoid resistance cases) and applied in cases where chloroquine-resistant strains are reported .

While the use of current drugs have reduced the death rate, the research and development of a 100% effective malaria therapy, as well as the search for a vaccine development, remains an issue of global concern [33].

CONFLICT OF INTEREST

The authors confirm that they have no conflict of interest to declare for this publication.

ACKNOWLEDGEMENTS

Declared none.

REFERENCES

[1] Cholewiński M, Derda M, Hadaś E. Parasitic diseases in humans transmitted by vectors. Ann Parasitol 2015; 61(3): 137-57.
[PMID: 26568987]

[2] Centers for disease Control and Prevention [homepage on the internet]. Atlanta. Available from: http://www.cdc.gov/malaria/about/biology/

[3] National Institute of Allergy and Infectious Diseases [homepage on the internet] . Bethesda, Maryland [updated th January, 2016]. Available at: https://www.niaid.nih.gov/topics/Malaria/Pages/lifecycle.aspx

[4] Medicines for Malaria Venture. [homepage on the internet] . USA: [updated, 2016]. Available at: http://www.mmv.org/sites/default/files/uploads/images/malaria_and_medicines/posters_parasitelife

[5] Malaria-West Nile Virus [homepage on the internet] . Greece. University of Thessaly. [updated, 2016]. Available at: http://www.malwest.gr/enus/malaria/informationforhealthcareprofessionals/plasmodiumlifecycle.aspx

[6] 6. World Health Organization Media Centre. [homepage on the internet]. 2010. USA: [updated August]. 2010. Fact Sheets on malaria. Available at: http://www.who.int/mediacentre/factsheets/fs094/en/index.html and http://www.who.int/features/factfiles/malaria/en/index.html

[7] Ministry of Health, Government of Southern Sudan. Prevention and treatment guidelines for primary health centres and hospitals [homepage on the internet] Sudan. [updated 2006]. Available at: http://www.southernsudanmedicaljournal.com/assets/files/misc/SS_Treatment_Guidelines07.pdf

[8] Warrell DA, Gilles HM, Eds. Essential Malariology. 4th ed. 2002; pp. 236-49. Chapter 10

[9] Hartman TK, Rogerson SJ, Fischer PR. The impact of maternal malaria on newborns. The Annals of Tropical Pediatrics. Int Child Health 2010; 30: 271-82.

[10] Al-Bari MA. Chloroquine analogues in drug discovery: new directions of uses, mechanisms of actions and toxic manifestations from malaria to multifarious diseases. J Antimicrob Chemother 2015; 70(6): 1608-21.
[http://dx.doi.org/10.1093/jac/dkv018] [PMID: 25693996]

[11] Achan J, Talisuna AO, Erhart A, *et al.* Quinine, an old anti-malarial drug in a modern world: role in the treatment of malaria. Malar J 2011; 10: 144.
[http://dx.doi.org/10.1186/1475-2875-10-144] [PMID: 21609473]

[12] Silva GN, Rezende LC, Emery FS, Gosmann G, Gnoatto SC. Natural and semi synthetic antimalarial compounds: emphasis on the terpene class. Mini Rev Med Chem 2015; 15(10): 809-36.
[http://dx.doi.org/10.2174/1389557515666150101101519] [PMID: 25553426]

[13] National Center for Biotechnology. Information PubChem Compound Database; CID=3034034 2016. [cited 31st Jan 2016]. Available at: https://pubchem.ncbi.nlm.nih.gov/coumpound/3034034

[14] ChemAxon [Computer program]. Intuitive Application and API for chemical sketching visualization and data exploration 2016. Version 16.1.25.0. 2016

[15] National Center for Biotechnology. Information PubChem Compound Database; CID=2719 2016. [cited 31st Jan 2016]. Available at: https://pubchem.ncbi.nlm.nih.gov/coumpound/2719

[16] National Center for Biotechnology. Information PubChem Compound Database; CID=68827 2016. Available at: https://pubchem.ncbi.nlm.nih.gov/coumpound/68827

[17] National Center for Biotechnology. 2016. [cited 31st Jan 2016]. Available at: https://pubchem.ncbi.nlm.nih.gov/coumpound/4908 (cited 31st Jan 2016)

[18] Ploypradith P. Development of artemisinin and its structurally simplified trioxane derivatives as antimalarial drugs. Acta Trop 2004; 89(3): 329-42. [http://dx.doi.org/10.1016/j.actatropica.2003.10.006] [PMID: 14744559]

[19] Barmade MA, Murumkar PR, Sharma MK, Shingala KP, Giridhar RR, Yadav MR. Discovery of anti-malarial agents through application of *in silico* studies. Comb Chem High Throughput Screen 2015; 18(2): 151-87. [http://dx.doi.org/10.2174/1386207318666141229125852] [PMID: 25543680]

[20] CDC. Treatment of malaria (Guidelines for clinicians). Centers for Diseases Control and Prevention 2013.

[21] WHO. Guidelines for the treatment of malaria World Health Organization . 3rd ed., Geneva 2015.

[22] Bijker EM, Bastiaens GJ, Teirlinck AC, *et al.* Protection against malaria after immunization by chloroquine prophylaxis and sporozoites is mediated by preerythrocytic immunity. Proc Natl Acad Sci USA 2013; 110(19): 7862-7. [http://dx.doi.org/10.1073/pnas.1220360110] [PMID: 23599283]

[23] Shi C, Li H, Yang Y, Hou L. Anti-inflammatory and immunoregulatory functions of artemisinina and its derivates. Mediators Inflamm 2015; ID: 435713

[24] Rolling T, Wichmann D, Schmiedel S, Burchard GD, Kluge S, Cramer JP. Artesunate versus quinine in the treatment of severe imported malaria: comparative analysis of adverse events focussing on delayed haemolysis. Malar J 2013; 12: 241. [http://dx.doi.org/10.1186/1475-2875-12-241] [PMID: 23855745]

[25] Bruxvoort K, Goodman C, Kachur SP, Schellenberg D. How patients take malaria treatment: a systematic review of the literature on adherence to antimalarial drugs. PLoS One 2014; 9(1): e84555. [http://dx.doi.org/10.1371/journal.pone.0084555] [PMID: 24465418]

[26] Ibraheem ZO, Majid RA, Noor SM, Sedik HM, Basir R. Role of different Pfcrt and Pfmdr-1 in conferring resistance to antimalarial drugs in Plasmodium falciparum. Malar Res Treat 2014; 2014: 950424.

[27] Maguire JD, Sumawinata IW, Masbar S, *et al.* Chloroquine-resistant Plasmodium malariae in south Sumatra, Indonesia. Lancet 2002; 360(9326): 58-60. [http://dx.doi.org/10.1016/S0140-6736(02)09336-4] [PMID: 12114045]

[28] Ecker A, Lehane AM, Clain J, Fidock DA. PfCRT and its role in antimalarial drug resistance. Trends Parasitol 2012; 28(11): 504-14.

[http://dx.doi.org/10.1016/j.pt.2012.08.002] [PMID: 23020971]

[29] World Health Organization. [homepage on the internet] . USA. [updated 2015]. Available at: http://www.who.int/features/factfiles/malaria/es/

[30] Gamo FJ. Antimalarial drug resistance: new treatments options for *Plasmodium*. Drug Discov Today Technol 2014; 11: 81-8. [http://dx.doi.org/10.1016/j.ddtec.2014.03.002] [PMID: 24847657]

[31] Dondorp AM, Nosten F, Yi P, *et al.* Artemisinin resistance in *Plasmodium falciparum* malaria. N Engl J Med. 2009; 361: pp. (5)455-67. [http://dx.doi.org/10.1056/NEJMoa0808859] [PMID: 19641202]

[32] Sibley CH. Understanding drug resistance in malaria parasites: basic science for public health. Mol Biochem Parasitol 2014; 195(2): 107-14. [http://dx.doi.org/10.1016/j.molbiopara.2014.06.001] [PMID: 24927641]

[33] Torrús D, Carranza C, Manuel Ramos J, *et al.* [Microbiological diagnosis of imported malaria]. Enferm Infecc Microbiol Clin 2015; 33 (Suppl. 2): 40-6. [http://dx.doi.org/10.1016/S0213-005X(15)30014-8] [PMID: 26320995]

CHAPTER 5

Update on Advances in Plant-based Antimalarial Drug Discovery

Pius S. Fasinu[1,*], **Ilias Muhammad**[1] and **Larry A. Walker**[1,2]

[1] *National Center for Natural Products Research, Research Institute of Pharmaceutical Sciences, School of Pharmacy, University of Mississippi, University MS, 38677, USA*

[2] *Department of BioMolecular Sciences, University of Mississippi, University MS, 38677, USA*

Abstract: Malaria remains one of the major infectious diseases with high morbidity and mortality in developing and under-developed countries of the world. Although readily curable, the development of resistance by the malaria parasite especially *Plasmodium falciparum*, to existing antimalarials necessitates the need for continuous search for new antimalarial drugs. Several approaches have been adopted in this search including those based on natural products, particularly medicinal plants and herbs. As exemplified in the discovery of quinine and artemisinin, there has been intensified effort in the search of safe and efficacious plant-based antimalarial compounds. This search has yielded moderate success. The current chapter highlights the most promising plant-based drug discovery success with particular emphasis on studies that have reached some advanced clinical stages. With many plant-based compounds exerting antimalarial activities through multiple mechanisms, it is expected that further studies will complement current research efforts towards successful antimalarial drug discovery and development.

Keywords: Artemisinin, Chloroquine, Drug discovery, Herbal medicine, Malaria, Natural products, Plant-derived drugs, *Plasmodium falciparum*, Quinine, Reversed pharmacology.

* **Corresponding author Pius S Fasinu:** National Center for Natural Products Research, University of Mississippi, University MS, 38677, USA; Tel: 1-662-915-1005; Fax: 1-662-915-1006; E-mail: psfasinu@olemiss.edu.

Norma Rivera (Ed.)

INTRODUCTION

Malaria has remained a major health challenge in several countries of the world and according to the World Health Organization (WHO) 2014 malaria statistics, 97 countries and territories of the world have ongoing malaria transmission with 3.3 billion people at risk, an estimated 198 million cases and 584000 deaths in 2013, 85% of who are children under 5 years old [1]. Pregnant women are among the group hardest hit by malaria prevalence, and made worse by limited drug choices. *Plasmodium falciparum*, the most virulent malaria parasite, has developed resistance to most of the available antimalarial drugs [2]. The current standard of treatment as recommended by WHO is artemisinin (ART)-based combination therapy (ACT) comprising artemisinin (or its derivative) in combination with another antimalarial usually an arylamino alcohol or 4-aminoquinoline [3]. Increasing reports of malaria resistance to ACTs, occasioned by delayed cure of parasitaemia and fever symptoms in patients in Southeast Asia and Africa, is a current threat which can only be offset, in the long term, by the discovery of new antimalarial drugs [4, 5].

There is a general consensus on what an ideal antimalarial drug should be. Apart from effectiveness against malaria and demonstration of superiority over existing drugs, an acceptable antimalarial drug should exert actions *via* novel mechanisms that will safeguard against parasite resistance. More important, however, is the economic factor. Malaria is prevalent in developing and under-developed countries of the world. The resource limitation implies that effective drugs should be affordable in order to reach the target population and enhance treatment compliance. Several approaches have been adopted in antimalarial drug discovery and development. These include optimization of therapy through existing drugs. This generally involves the combination of unrelated antimalarial drugs to explore multiple mechanisms of action against the parasite as seen in various marketed antimalarial formulations [6]. Another approach is the development of analogs of existing antimalarial drugs with the purpose of improving efficacy and safety. This approach has been successful with, for example, the development of several aminoquinolines based on quinine [7]. And yet another approach is the search for bioactives and lead compounds from natural products.

The historical relevance of plant-derived compounds in antimalarial chemotherapy suggests that, despite the limited success in recent times, successful antimalarial drug discoveries are possible from botanicals. Natural products present an endless source of potential new pharmacophores upon which synthetic analogues and modifications can be based. Several novel compounds are yet undiscovered from plants many of which, like quinine and ART, are not only therapeutically active on their own, but provide new leads into synthetic antimalarial drug discovery. The high perception of safety of natural products by health consumers, often founded on centuries of traditional use, has made natural products more appealing and acceptable as potential sources of therapeutic agents. While this perception seems to favor popular trust in herbal products, it should be noted that phytochemicals are not always free of toxicity and safety data are required before regulatory approval.

In most malaria-endemic communities, there is anecdotal evidence of antimalarial activity for a wide range of ethnobotanical remedies. This provides the basis for initial antimalarial screenings and bioassay-guided isolation and purification in drug discovery [8]. Additionally, there is some commitment to research and preservation of traditionally useful ethnobotanical resources in malaria-endemic countries [8] especially in Africa. Apart from global climate change, which poses a threat to expand malaria towards the areas of high elevation in Africa and South Asia, as well as the resultant climate change due to rapid urbanization and other human activities has been recognized as responsible for increasing the number of valuable traditional plants going into extinction [9]. These factors highlight the urgency and favorable considerations in antimalarial drug discovery focusing on natural products to provide leads.

In this chapter, an update on plant-based antimalarial drug discovery efforts is provided with emphasis on those lead compounds and products that have reached some stages of assessment in humans since after the discovery of quinine. A brief description of the discovery of the prototypical natural product antimalarial drugs quinine and ART is included to provide historical perspective of the relationship between malaria drug discovery and phytochemicals.

Historical Relationship Between Phytochemicals and Antimalarial Drug Discovery

Historically, antimalarial chemotherapy is strongly linked to traditional medicine. There has been a consistent pattern of isolation of active antimalarial entities from natural products followed by chemical and pharmaceutical modifications to arrive at equally or more effective drugs. Quinine, the very first antimalarial drug, was isolated and purified in 1882 from the bark of *Cinchona* species, a plant with long history of use in the treatment of malaria fever. Quinine provided the structural backbone for the discovery and synthesis of other antimalarial drugs including the 4-aminoquinolines and the amino-alcohols such as amodiaquine, chloroquine and mefloquine; and the 8-aminoquinoline – primaquine [10]. These quinolines have been the mainstay of malaria treatment for several decades. The further discovery of the naphthoquinone, lapachol, from *Tabebuia avellanedae* (Bignoniaceae) as one of the active chemical constituents provided the basis for the discovery of atovaquone, an antimalarial still used for prophylaxis [11].

The current WHO recommended treatment of *P. falciparum* malaria is based on ART. First isolated and characterized from the leaves of the Chinese plant, *Artemisia annua* in 1971, artemisinin has formed the basis for the development of highly effective antimalarial drugs [12].

Finding Potential Antimalarial Agents from Natural Products

a. Influence of Modern High-Throughput Assay Technologies on Drug Discovery Efforts

Over the past decade, high throughput techniques have been developed to enhance the screening of chemical compounds against various infective organisms including parasites. These technological advances have greatly facilitated the investigation of traditional antimalarials in the search of chemical leads.

Following the first report of the continuous *in vitro* cultivation of the human malaria parasite, *P. falciparum*, in 1976 [13] microplate assay techniques were developed in which parasite growth can be monitored through the uptake of [^{3}H] hypoxanthine by infected red blood cells. This allows the assessment of the effect of test compounds on the cultivated parasites [14]. Further, acolorimetric method, designed to overcome the necessity of radiolabeled substrates represents a recent advance which has improved screening efficiency and saved time and resources. In this method, 3-acetylpyridine adenine dinucleotide (APAD) is used as the substrate for plasmodial lactate dehydrogenase, whereby a dark blue color is produced as the parasite grows [15]. This allows results to be read without the aid of spectrophotometer, although such does allow for quantitative assessments of parasite growth. Other advances in assay methodologies include those developed to investigate liver stage parasites and gametocytes [16].

The complete sequencing of the genome of the malaria parasite has made a systematic analysis of all the essential genes possible. Due to advances in imaging and automation technology, assays for live malarial parasites inside host cells can now be performed in large-scale formats including 384 or 1536 well formats, a development that is being utilized in screening thousands of herbal extracts, phytochemicals and synthetic compounds for antimalarial potentials [17]. The utilization of these high throughput techniques has led to considerable success in identifying a variety of potential antimalarial compounds from natural products. Cell-based screening, in addition to providing information on the lethal effect of the test compound on the parasite offers simultaneous information on the cell permeability and toxicity when for example, parasites in human blood cells are used. High throughput procedures for the fractionation of plant products have been developed, and in combination with modern biological screening techniques, offer a convenient approach in the search for leads [18].

b. Drug Discovery and Development from Natural Products

Over time, the search for antimalarial drugs from natural products has been conducted in two ways. One approach is the indiscriminate *in vitro* screening of extract libraries from a wide range of natural sources, including plants, herbal products and marine resources. Potential antimalarial active compounds are then isolated for further studies including in animals and if suitable in humans (Fig. **1**). Success rate from this method has been very limited. The other approach involves the reliance on anecdotal evidence and ethno-pharmacological data from traditional antimalarial uses. It has been argued that this method may improve success rate. Also referred to as reverse-pharmacology, ethnobotany-based drug discovery starts with some evidence of activity in humans which is then followed by studies *in vitro* and in animals [19]. This method is considered more cost effective since it would be more expedient to have some activity confirmation of crude extracts before embarking on costly and extensive chemical isolation and characterization.

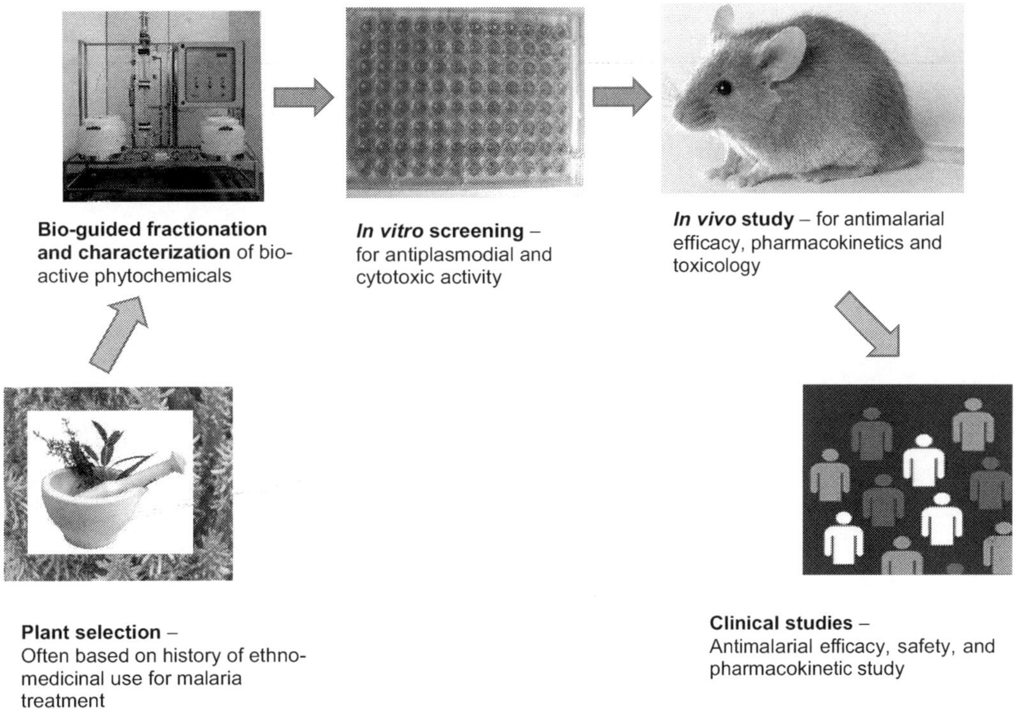

Fig. (1). Drug discovery process from botanicals including screening, bio-guided isolation and characterization of bioactive phytochemicals and confirmation of activity through preclinical and clinical studies.

In accordance with regulatory guidelines [19], studies must be conducted in humans, in addition to long history of traditional use of the test plant extract or herbal product, where side effects and toxicities are well documented. Generally, drugs discovery process from this approach tends to follow a pattern, often called reverse pharmacology (Fig. **2**) [19]. Features of reverse pharmacology approach to plant-based drug discovery can be summarized as follows:

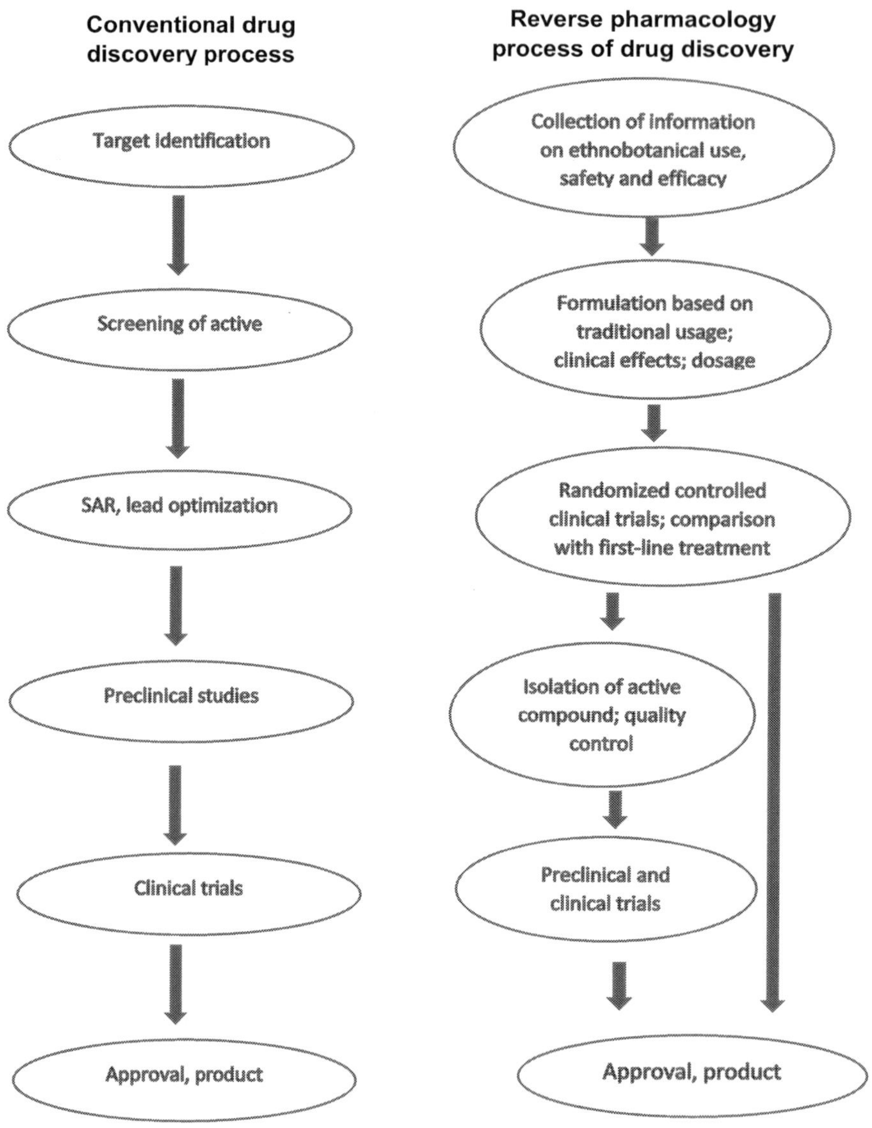

Fig. (2). Comparative schematic representation of the traditional drug discovery (often referred to as 'bench to the bedside') and reversed pharmacology drug discovery process (also known as 'clinic to laboratory' approach).

a. Reports and evidence of efficacy following a long history of use of the identified plant extract or herbal product; clinical assessment of the activity of the extracts in human subjects including cure of parasitemia, resolution of other symptoms like fever or the ability to boost body's immunity against the parasite; analysis of human tissue samples to confirm activity *ex vivo* and elucidate possible mechanism of action.

b. A more mechanistic study *in vivo* using animal models where activity against different species of *Plasmodium* can be assessed; comparative responses in human and animal models.
c. *In vitro* assessment of the extracts against *Plasmodium* species in culture; assessment against the different stages of the parasite development including blood and liver stages; comparison of effective concentrations *in vitro* and in plasma.
d. Isolation and purification of the active phytochemicals; confirmation of activity retention after isolation and investigation of the presence of multiple active component in the crude extract.
e. Metabolism, pharmacokinetic, toxicological assessment and clinical trials of isolated phytochemical.
f. Pharmaceutical development.

From Quinine to Several Quinolines

Quinine is the antimalarial principle isolated from the bark of Cinchona species (Rubiaceae). It was the first effective treatment for *P. falciparum* malaria. Before quinine (Fig. **3**) was extracted, purified and named by Pierre Joseph Pelletier and Joseph Caventou in 1820, fine powder was made from dried cinchona bark and mixed into a liquid before being taken [10]. Quinine henceforth replaced the crude bark and remained the only effective antimalarial drug until its synthetic derivatives were available in the 1940s. Other alkaloids isolated from cinchona bark with antimalarial property include quinidine (now clinically used for the management of cardiac arrhythmias), cinchonine and cinchonidine. One of the early clinical trials conducted between 1866 and 1868 in 3600 patients to assess the antimalarial efficacies of the four cinchona alkaloids showed that all four were effective with cure rates greater than 98%. The efficacies of these four alkaloids were evaluated in one of the earliest clinical trials. With the main outcome measure of "cessation of febrile paroxysms", all four alkaloids were found to be comparable, with cure rates of > 98% [20].

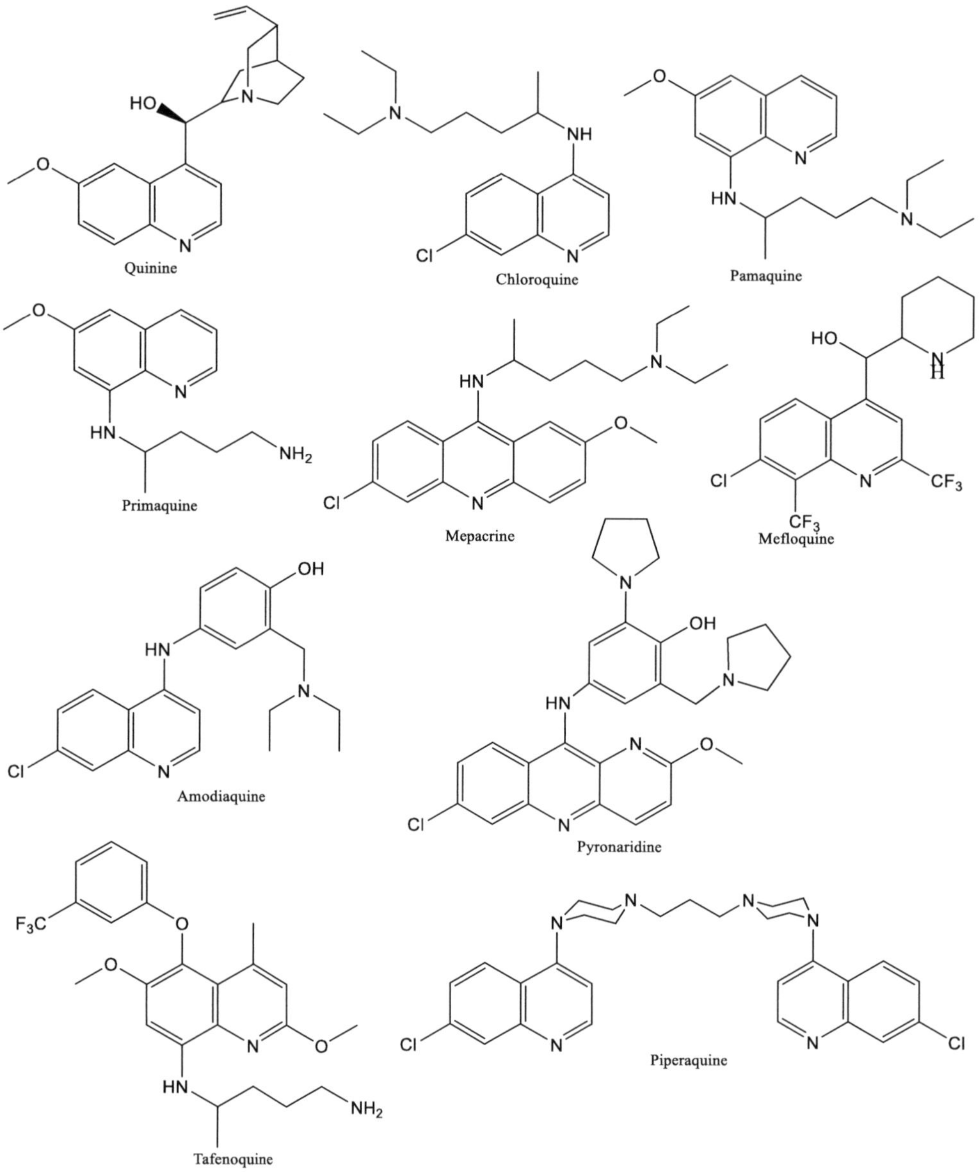

Fig. (3). Quinine from *Cinchona* species and its various natural derivatives and synthetic analogs.

Until the 1920s, quinine was the mainstay of malaria treatment and provided the chemical and structural basis for the synthesis of more effective antimalarial drugs especially chloroquine which was extensively used and popularized in the 1940s. After decades of extensive use, resistance of P. falciparum to chloroquine crept in and quinine again, returned to clinical use especially in the treatment of uncomplicated malaria. For example, the 2010 WHO guidelines recommend quinine in combination with doxycycline, tetracycline or clindamycin as second-line option for the treatment for uncomplicated malaria; as well as in combination with clindamycin for malaria treatment in the first trimester of pregnancy [21].

Quinine, one of the most serendipitous medical discoveries in history, has remained a major antimalarial drug after four decades. Till date, the basic structure of quinine is still being explored in the development of various quinolines (Fig. **3**). Recent publications are available for a more extensive reviews of the role of quinine in antimalarial drug discovery [22, 23].

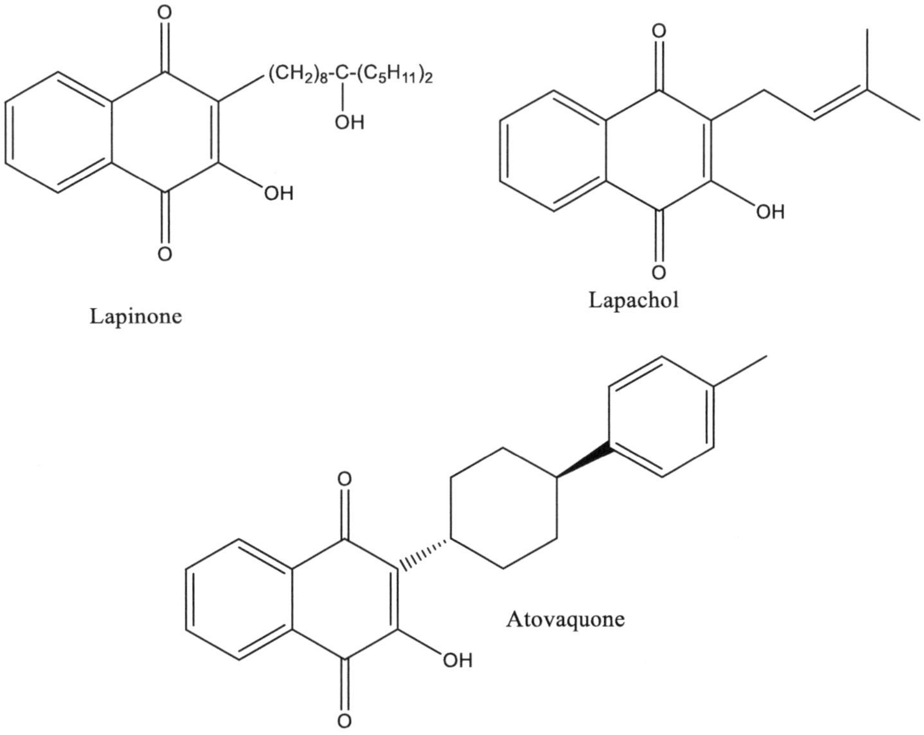

Fig. (4). Chemical structures of lapinone, lapachol and atovaquone.

Atovaquone

Atovaquone is a product of chemical modification and optimization of lapinone, a derivative of lapachol (Fig. **4**). Lapachol, a naphthoquinone used in the treatment of malaria and fever was first isolated from the stem bark of *Tabebuia avellanedae* (Bignoniaceae) in 1882 [24, 25]. From earlier studies, lapachol demonstrated a very weak curative activity in *P. zophurae* -infected ducks. It provided the lead for a more active derivative, lapinone which showed activity against *P. vivax* in human subjects [26]. A further chemical modification yielded atovaquone (Fig. **4**) which is still in clinical use (Malarone®) for prophylaxis against *P. falciparum* malaria. Lapachol and its derivatives inhibit electron transport in the parasite. While atovaquone is a reliable drug today for preventing malaria infection, it might have been impossible to discover it if not for the lead provided by phytochemicals from *T. avellanedae* [27].

Artemisinin and the Endoperoxides

Artemisinin is a sesquiterpene endoperoxide isolated and characterized from sweet wormwood, *Artemisia annua* (Asteraceae) through deliberate antimalarial research efforts of a consortium of Chinese scientists, supported by the Chinese government, in early seventies. ART is effective against all stages – sexual and asexual – of the parasite development. It activates free radicals in the presence of free ferrous iron which is produced in erythrocytes by the digestion of hemoglobin by the parasite. ART has limited clinical utility due to its short plasma half-life, poor solubility and bioavailability.

Efforts to improve on the properties of artemisinin yielded the first generation ART derivatives (Fig. **5**). Of these derivatives, dihydroartemisinin, the product of the reduction of ART in the presence of sodium borohydride, is the most potent, by over six times compared to ART, against malarial parasites in *in vitro* models. Other first generation analogs of ART include the ether derivatives – artemether and arteether which are oil soluble and well absorbed after intramuscular administration; and artesunate which is water soluble and can be given intravenously. ART and its first generation analogs have very good safety profiles and fast onset of action making them effective in cerebral malaria. They are effective in the management of uncomplicated and severe *P. falciparum* malaria, as well as blood stage infections of *P. vivax*.

Through the studies of the structure-activity relationships of ART and in order to improve its pharmacological activity, several endoperoxides have been synthesized. Modifications on the 1,2,3-trioxane ring structure of artemisinin have also been made. The earlier forms include modification at the C-10 position of the dihydroartemisinin giving the simple ester or ether derivatives which demonstrated major improvement in efficacy and solubility over ART. Further attempts were made to obtain new antimalarial drugs through C-10 or C-14 substitutions. In all these, it has been shown that the 1,2,3-trioxane ring on its own is not sufficient for antimalarial activity, that the endoperoxide is the essential pharmacophoric unit [28 - 31].

Through this effort, OZ277 (Fig. **5**), a promising cyclic peroxide has been produced with *in vitro* antimalarial activity [32]. Others include fully synthetic and simplified peroxides such as fenozan B07 [33, 34], the dispiro tetraoxanes [35], tricyclic simplified 1,2,4-trioxanes [36] and simple endoperoxide analogues [37]. So far, OZ277, which has demonstrated more potent activity and stability than ART *in vitro*, has received the most attention towards antimalarial drug development [38].

Generally, ART has provided a lead into the discovery of sesquiterpene endoperoxides, an unusual class of structures that are very specific towards malaria parasite irrespective of the carrier structures, and without causing significant side effects or damage to human cells.

Yingzhaosu, a peroxy moiety-containing sesquiterpene is the active antimalarial constituent isolated from the traditional Chinese antimalarial plant, *Artabotrys uncinatus* (L.) Merr. (Annonaceae), called Yingzhao. It has a unique structure made of a dioxabicyclo(3,3,1)-nonane ring to which a dihydroxy-olefinic side chain is attached. It has been synthesized [39].

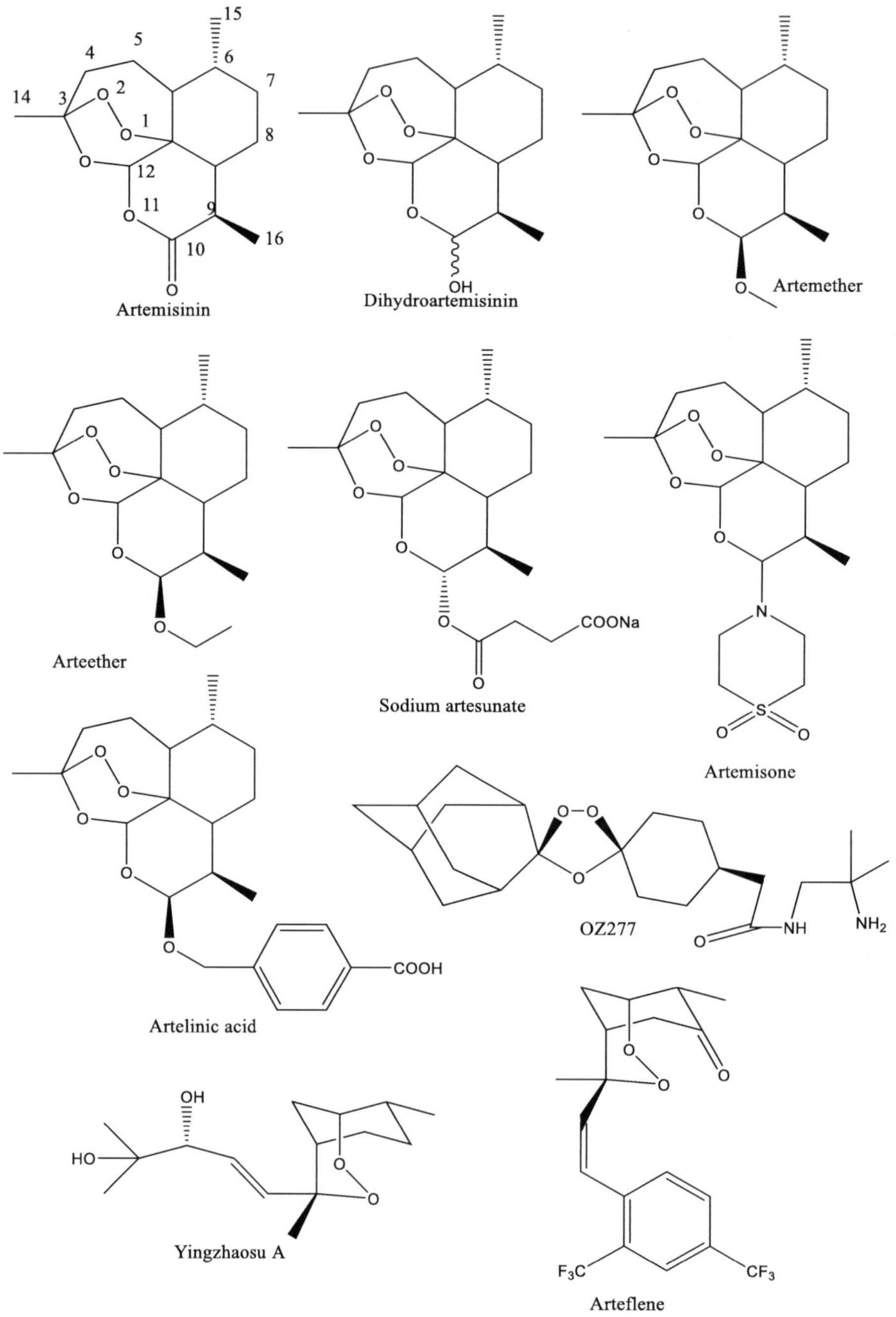

Fig. (5). Structure of artemisinin and its natural and synthetic derivatives, and other endoperoxides.

Based on the structure of Yingzhaosu, a synthetic peroxide, Ro 42-1611 (arteflene) was developed (Fig. **5**). Arteflene was a promising antimalarial compound that progressed substantially in development. It demonstrated *in vivo* activity 4-5 fold higher after parenteral than after oral administration in mice due to poor oral bioavailability [40]. Arteflene was well tolerated in man as demonstrated by a single ascending dose, double-blind, placebo-controlled trial in nine healthy male volunteers where no serious adverse effect was observed [41]. After a successful phase II trial, 80% of patients (N=30; parasitaemia > 5000/ml; temperature 37.7 -39.8ºC; aged 12 -42) treated with a single 25 mg/kg arteflene dose, were parasite free by day 7 [42]. Arteflene showed high clinical cure rates with 70% of all patients free of all signs and symptoms after 24 hours of administration. Arteflene was compared against mefloquine in a phase 3, open-labeled, randomized clinical trial for the treatment of uncomplicated malaria in children [43]. Although it cleared fever slightly faster than mefloquine, arteflene did not demonstrate superiority to mefloquine in terms of parasite clearance which led to the discontinuation of its development [43].

Cryptolepine and Related Quinolines

Cryptolepine (5-methyl indolo[2,3b]-quinoline) is a naturally occurring indoloquinoline alkaloid first isolated from the roots of *Cryptolepis sanguinolenta* (Apocyanaceae), an African plant, whose extracts have been traditionally used for the cure of malaria [44, 45]. Other alkaloids latter isolated from this plant includes quindoline, cryptospirolepine and isocryptolepine (Fig. **6**). Cryptolepine has demonstrated potent antimalarial activity in preclinical evaluations [46 - 49].

An herbal tea of *Cryptolepis sanguinolenta* formulated by a local Ghanaian pharmaceutical company and named Phyto-Laria® was clinically evaluated for antimalarial activity. In a prospective descriptive open trial conducted in 44 symptomatic subjects with uncomplicated malaria, Bugyei *et al.* (2010) [50] administered extracts of a 2.5 g tea bag formulation containing powdered root of the herb to each patients three times daily for five days. The authors reported the clearance of parasitemia in 50% of the patients after 72 hours, and in all subjects by the 7th day; in addition to the clearance of symptoms - fever, chills, nausea and vomiting – in all patients by the third day. These findings suggest that cryptolepine could be an effective antimalarial drug.

Through structural modifications, several derivatives of cryptolepine have been synthesized and evaluated for enhanced efficacy with the most promising being 11-(4-piperidinamino)cryptolepine HCl (Fig. **6**), which showed a potent *in vitro* activity (IC_{50} = 44 nM) against *P. falciparum* with the least cytotoxicity [51, 52].

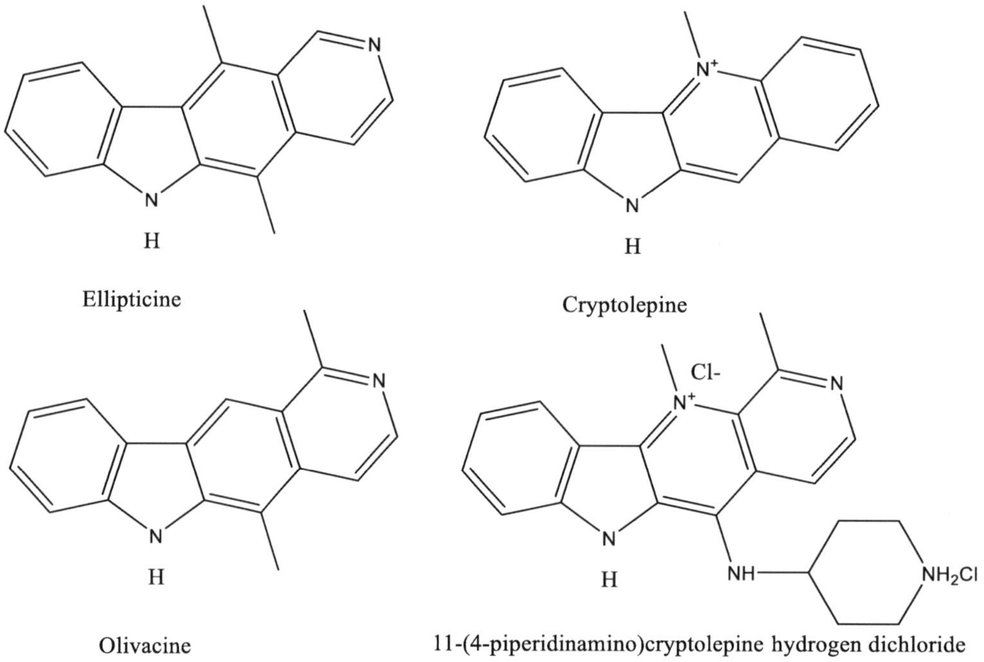

Fig. (6). Structures of antimalarial compounds ellipticine, cryptolepine, olivacine and 11-(4-piperidinamino) cryptolepine HCl.

Strictosamide and its Derivatives from *Nauclea Pobeguinii*

Strictosamide Fig. (**7**) is the active constituent isolated from the stem bark of *N. pobeguinii* (Rubiaceae), a plant whose decoction is traditionally used for the treatment of uncomplicated malaria in Africa [53]. Other alkaloids including angustine, angustoline, 3,14-dihydro-angustine, naufoline, nauclefine and O-acetyl-angustoline, have been isolated from the plant.

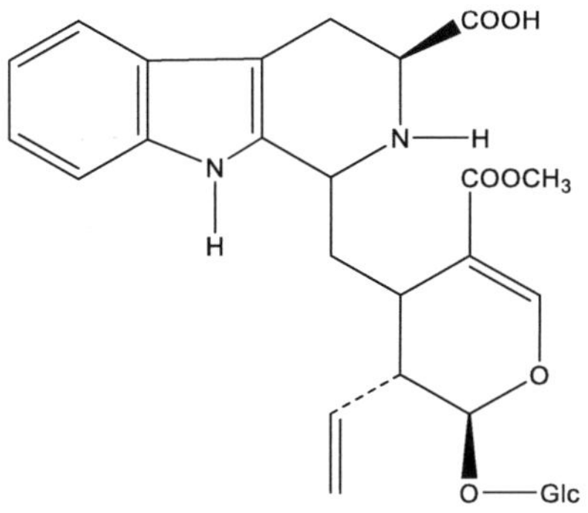

5(*S*)-5-carboxystrictosidine

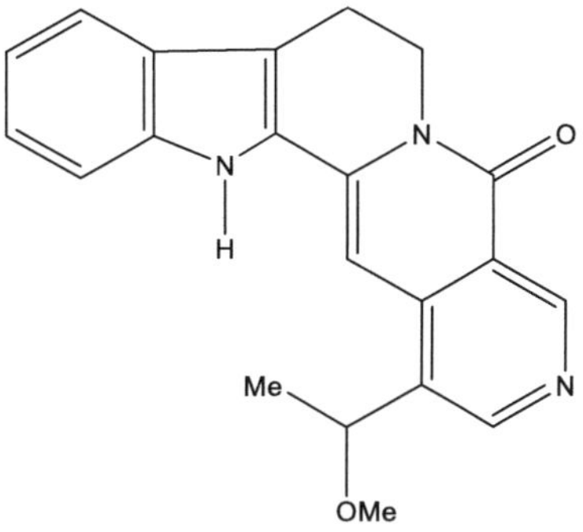

19-*O*-methylangustoline

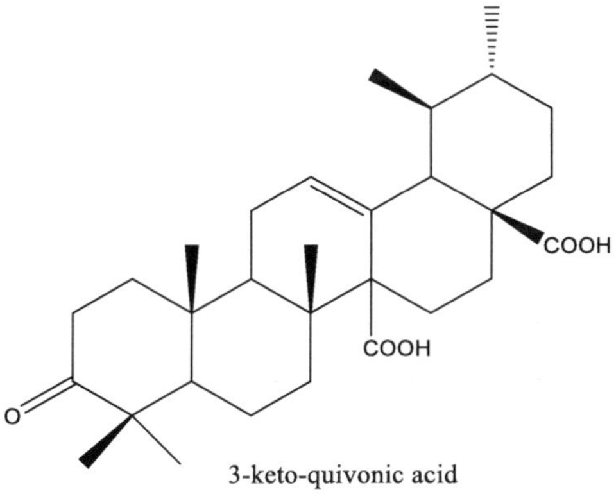

3-keto-quivonic acid

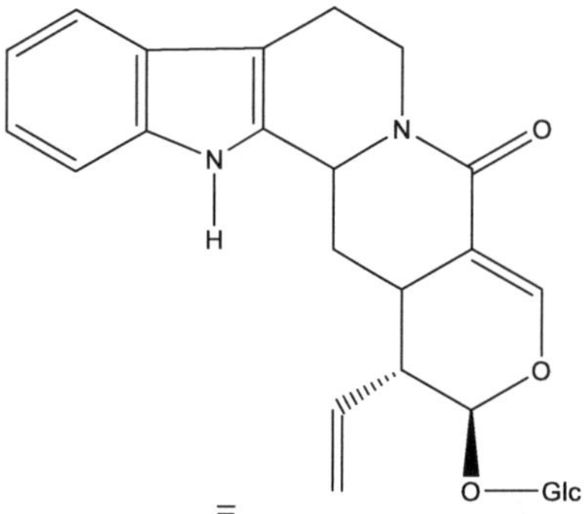

Strictosamide

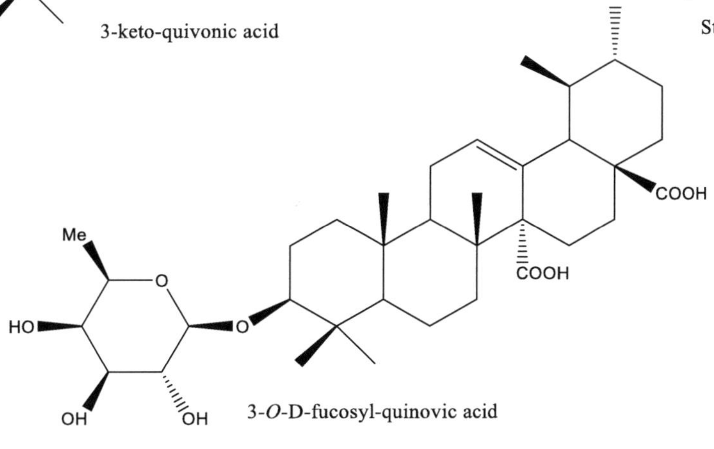

3-*O*-D-fucosyl-quinovic acid

Fig. (7). Structures of compounds isolated from the stem bark of *Nauclea pobeguinii.*

In a phase I clinical study, PR 259 CT1, an 80% ethanolic extract of the stem bark of *N. pobeguinii* characterized and quantified to contain 5.6% strictosamide and formulated into 500 mg capsules was administered to 15 healthy subjects (two capsules, three times daily for seven days) [54]. The absence of clinically significant adverse effects of PR 259 CT1 at the given dose, in addition to the long history of traditional use, suggests that the products may not pose major safety concerns. In a further phase IIA study to assess the antimalarial efficacy of PR 259 CT1, an open cohort of eleven adult patients diagnosed with uncomplicated malaria were administered with a three-times-daily regimen of two 500 mg capsules for three days, followed by a one 500 mg capsule three times daily for the next four days. Authors reported that all but one patient were cleared of parasitemia and associated symptoms of fever by the fourth day [55]. Side effects were minimal and self-resolving similar to those observed in phase I study. Using the same dose regimen in a phase IIB single blind prospective trial in 65 patients diagnosed with uncomplicated malaria, PR 259 CT1 was as effective as artesunate-amodiaquine combination, the standard antimalarial regimen in Congo, where the study was conducted [56]. Additionally, less side effects were attributed to the test drug.

PR 259 CT1 is one of the very promising antimalarial standardized extracts awaiting further development and regulatory approval for clinical use. Strictosamide is also expected to provide a structural lead for synthetic antimalarial drugs for optimal activity, especially after its mechanism of antimalarial action has been elucidated.

Argemone Mexicana and its Chemical Constituents

Extracts and decoctions of *Argemone mexicana* (Papaveraceae) have been used as traditional medicine for the treatment of malaria. Principal compounds isolated and associated with antimalarial activity include allocryptopine, berberine and protopine (Fig. **8**). Traditional preparations of *A. mexicana* are government-approved for the treatment of malaria in Mali [57].

In a prospective and dose-escalating clinical trial conducted by Willcox *et al.* in Mali, decoctions of *A. mexicana* were administered to a total of 80 subjects with symptoms of malaria and *P. falciparum* parasitaemia >2000/µl [57]. Subjects who were administered the remedy twice daily for seven days had the highest proportion (73%) of adequate clinical response (ACR). The preparation was well tolerated with only minor side effects observed. In furtherance to this finding, the authors conducted a comparable study in 301 patients with uncomplicated malaria using the *A. mexicana* decoctions and artesunate-amodiaquine. After 28 days, second-line antimalarial treatment was not required for 89% of the patients who took *A. mexicana* compared to 95% in artesunate-amodiaquine group [58]. While these findings have led to official approval of the decoctions of *A. mexicana* for the treatment of malaria in Mali, along with traditional use in several other African countries, further research is necessary to explore the phytochemistry of the constituents for structure-activity relationship and optimization *via* synthetic analogs, if necessary.

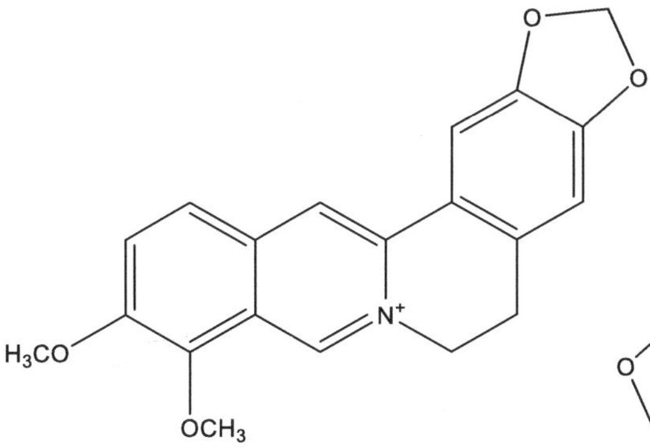

Berberine

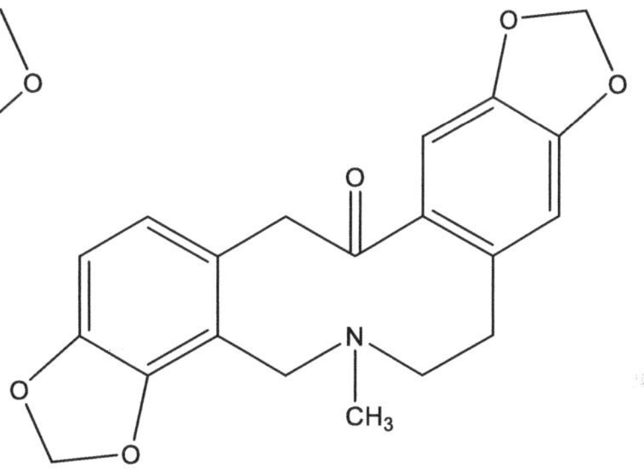

Protopine

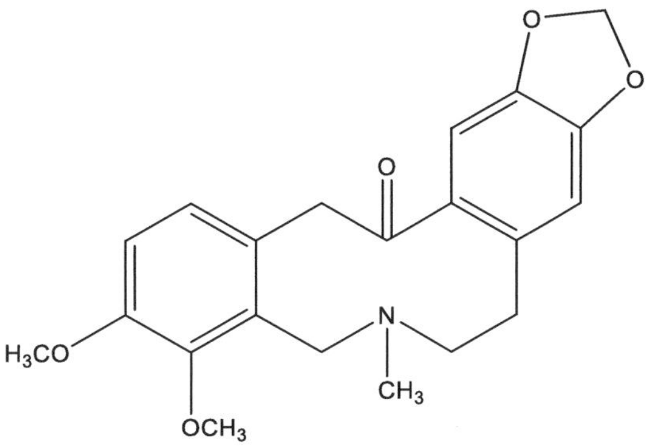

Allocryptopine

Fig. (8). Chemical structures of bio-active alkaloids from *Argemone mexicana*.

Vernodalin and its Analogs

Extracts of the leaves, root or whole plant of *Vernonia amygdalina* Del. (Compositae), a shrub widely found throughout Africa and often cultivated as a vegetable, is one of the most commonly used traditional medicine for the treatment of malaria in Africa [59 - 61]. The long history of nutritional consumption of the leaves of *V. amygdalina* suggests its safety in humans. A toxicity study in which rats were fed with food made up of 75% of the leaves of *V. amygdalina* for 65 days reported no signs of toxicity [62]. Studies *in vitro* and in animal models have confirmed antiplasmodial effects of the extracts of *V. amygdalina* [63, 64].

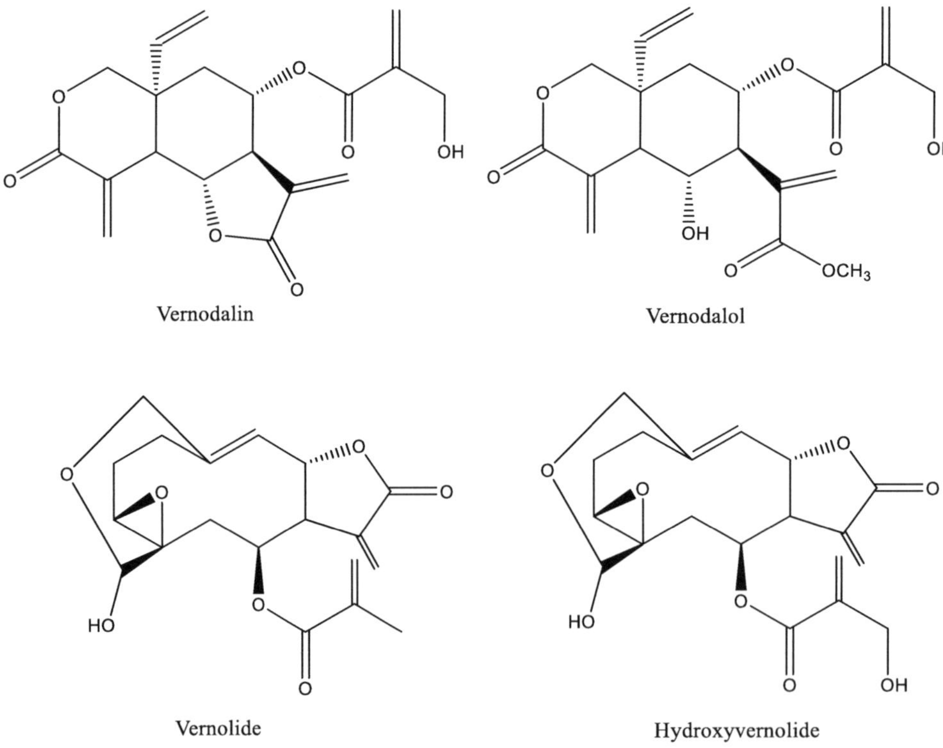

Fig. (9). Structures of sesquiterpene lactones from *Vernonia amygdalina*.

Several constituents have been isolated from *V. amygdalina*, including sesquiterpene lactones, namely vernodalin, vernolide, hydroxyvernolide, and vernodalol (Fig. **9**), which have some chemical similarities with sesquiterpenoid artemisinin, as well as steroidal glucosides, including vernoniosides A1-A4, and B1-B3, which give the plant its characteristic bitter taste. Vernodalin is reportedly the most abundant active compound in *V. amygdalina* [65].

In a multi-center clinical trial involving 33 human subjects in Uganda, the efficacy and safety of a 7-day, three times a day (every 8 hours) administration of the infusion of the leaves of *V. amygdalina* in the treatment of uncomplicated malaria were assessed. While the extract was well tolerated with no major side effect reported, only 67% of the subjects had adequate clinical response (ACR) by day 14. Out of those with ACR, only 32% had complete parasite clearance [66]. Although the study confirms the antimalarial potential of the extracts of *V. amygdalina* in agreement with long history of traditional use, it fails to demonstrate any superiority of the herb over existing antimalarial drugs. However, further studies on this herb are important as isolated compounds from it may be more effective than the crude extracts.

Febrifugine

Febrifugine (Fig. **10**), a quinazoline-type alkaloid is the active principle in the Chinese antimalarial plant *Dichroa febrifuga* (Saxifragaceae), *known locally as Ch'ang shan*. Extracts of the roots or the leaves have been used for centuries in the treatment of fever and malaria [67]. The effectiveness of febrifugine in the treatment of malaria has been reported several decades ago [68]. It was found to be effective against different species of *Plasmodium* and more active than quinine [69]. The widespread use of febrifugine was limited by reports of gastrointestinal toxicity which hampered its further development. However, febrifugine has been used as the lead compound towards the discovery of chemically related compounds with the potential for clinical utility in malaria treatment.

Modification to the febrifugine structure at the quinazoline ring, the linker, or the piperidine ring through structure-activity relationship has shown that the 4-quinazolinone moiety, the nitrogen atom of the piperidine ring, and the hydroxyl group are essential for the antimalarial activity. The absolute configuration of these functional groups is another important factor for activity. Modifications on the N3 side chain of the 4-quinazolinone ring did not improve antimalarial activity [70 - 73].

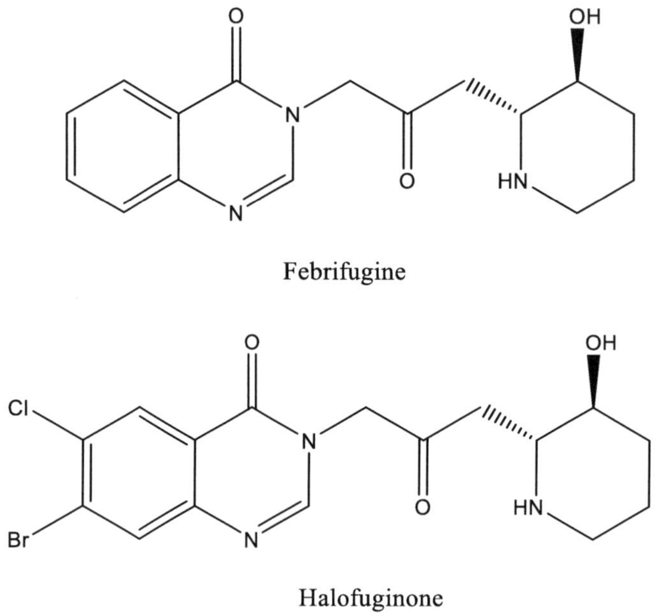

Fig. (10). Structures of febrifugine and halofuginone.

Of the several analogs of febrifugine synthesized and screened for antimalarial activity, halofuginone {7-bromo-6-chloro-3-[3 - l]-4(3H)-quinazolinone} (Fig. **6**) is the best known as it is used as antiprotozoal agent in cattle as well as additive in poultry feed for the prevention of coccidiosis [74, 75].

Halofuginone has shown activity against various strains of *Plasmodium* both *in vitro* and in animal models [76]. It is believed to hold strong antimalarial potential because of its capacity to attack the protozoa at its different stages of development, including sporozoites, trophozoites, and schizonts presenting the capability of radical cure and prevention of recrudescence [77, 78]. Molecularly, febrifugine and its analogs have been suggested to exert antimalarial activity through interaction with prolyl-tRNA synthetase in the parasite [79]. While halofuginone is been investigated for multiple therapeutic possibilities, not much has been done for its clinical evaluation in the treatment of malaria.

Others

In the past two decades, extracts of several hundreds of plant species have been assessed for antiplasmodial activity. Such plants generally include those that have histories of traditional use in malaria and related conditions. In many cases, pure compounds have been isolated from such extracts that show antiplasmodial activity. However, in most cases, adequate studies on these extracts and compounds have not yet been conducted. For the purpose of this write-up, emphasis has been laid on compounds that have reached some advanced stages of development typified by some clinical studies. It is hoped, however, that the large number of plant-based screenings being done in recent times hold the potential for some antimalarial drug discovery. For a more extensive report on the recent results on *in vitro* and *in vivo* antiplasmodial screening of traditionally used antimalarial extracts, some recent reviews are recommended [80 - 82]. A summary of major compounds isolated from a variety of plants, and which have demonstrated *in vitro* antiplasmodial activity against various strains *P. falciparum* with IC_{50} values below 10 μM is provided in Table **1**.

Table 1. Isolated compounds with moderate or potent *in vitro* activity against various strains of *P. falciparum*.

Class	Plant	Compound*	*P. falciparum* Strain Used	IC_{50} µM	Reference
Alkaloids	*Albizia gummifera*	Budmunchiamine, 6-hydroxybudmunchiamine, 5-normethylbudmunchiamine, 6-hydroxy-5-normethylbudmunchiamine, 9-normethylbudmunchiamine	CQ-sensitive (NF54) and CQ-resistant (ENT30)	0.18 - 0.33[a]	[83]
	Albizia schimperiana	5,14-Dimethylbudmunchiamine, 6-hydroxybudmunchiamine, 5-normethylbudmunchiamine, 6-hydroxy-5-normethylbudmunchiamine	CQ-sensitive (D6) and CQ-resistant (W2)	0.23 - 0.35[b]	[84]
	Cryptolepis sanguinolenta	Biscryptolepine	CQ-resistant (K1)	0.27	[85]
	Desmos rostrata	Discretine N-oxide, discretine, dehydrodiscretine	CQ-resistant (K1)	0.9 - 4.2	[86]
	Duguetia hadrantha	Hadranthine A, sampangine, 3-methoxysampangine	CQ-sensitive (D6) and CQ-resistant (W2)	0.31 - 0.4	[87]
	Funtumia, elastica	Holarrhetine, conessine, holarrhesine, isoconessimine	CQ-resistant (FcB1)	0.17 - 3.39	[88]
	Heimia salicifolia	Epi-lyfoline	CQ-sensitive (D6) and CQ-resistant (W2)	6.7	[89]
	Lycoris traubii	1-O-(30S)-hydroxybutanoyllycorine	CQ-sensitive and CQ-resistant	1.2	[90]
	Michelia figo	Magnolamine	CQ-resistant (K1) and CQ-sensitive (FCR3)	1.28	[91]

(Table 1) contd.....

Class	Plant	Compound[*]	*P. falciparum* Strain Used	IC_{50} μM	Reference
	Nauclea officinalis	Naucleofficine A	Isolate FCC1-HN	9.7	[92]
	Nauclea orientalis	Naucleaorine	CQ-sensitive (D6)	6.9	[93]
	Polyalthia cerasoides	Bidebiline	Multidrug-resistant (K1)	7.7	[94]
	Prosopis glandulosa	Prosopilosidine, prosopilosine, isoprosopilosine, isoprosopilosidine, juliprosopine	CQ-sensitive (D6) and CQ-resistant (W2)	0.061 - 0.95	[95]
	Pseudoxandra cuspidata	1S,1'R-rodiasine	CQ-resistant (FcB1-Columbia and FcM29-Cameroon) strains	1.14	[96]
	Psychotria klugii	Klugine, 7'-O-demethylisocephaeline, cephaeline, isocephaeline, emetine	CQ-sensitive (D6) and CQ-resistant (W2)	0.058 - 6.7	[97]
	Sarcococca hookeriana	Hookerianamide H and I, sarcovagine C, dictyophlebine	CQ-resistant (W2)	2.4 - 6.6	[98]
	Stephania rotunda	Dehydroroemerine	CQ-resistant (W2)	0.36[b]	[99]
	Strychnopsis thouarsii	Tazopsine, sinococuline	CQ-resistant (FCB1)	3.1 - 4.5	[100]
	Triclisia sacleuxii	Phaeanthine, N-methylapateline, 1,2-dehydroapateline,	CQ-sensitive (3D7) and CQ resistant (W2)	0.93 - 1.72	[101]

(Table 1) contd.....

Class	Plant	Compound*	*P. falciparum* Strain Used	IC_{50} µM	Reference
	Zanthoxylum flavum	Chelerythrine, acetonate	CQ-resistant (W2)	3.4	[102]
	Zanthoxylum flavum	Dihydrorutaecarpine	CQ-resistant (W2)	3.4	[102]
	Zanthoxylum rhoifolium	Dihydronitidine	CQ-resistant (FCB1)	4.9	[100]
	Zanthoxylum syncarpum	Syncarpamide	CQ-sensitive (D6) and CQ-resistant (W2)	4.2	[103]
	Ziziphus oenoplia	Ziziphine N and Q	CQ-resistant (W2)	5.9 - 6.4	[105]
Coumarins	*Phyllanthus niruri*	1-O-galloyl-6-O-luteoyl-a-D-glucose	Multidrug-resistant (K1)	2.21	[105]
	Zanthoxylum flavum	Isoimperatorin,	CQ-resistant (W2)	2.7	[102]

(Table 1) contd.....

Class	Plant	Compound*	*P. falciparum* Strain Used	IC_{50} µM	Reference
Flavonoids and flavonoid derivatives	*Artocarpus altilis*	Cycloartocarpin, artocarpin, chaplashin, morusin, cudraflavone B, artonin E, and artobiloxanthone	Multidrug-resistant (K1)	4 - 9.9	[106]
	Artocarpus champeden	Artocarpones and B, artonin A artoindonesianin R heterophyllin, heteroflavanone C artoindonesianin	3D7 clone	0.001 - 1.3	[107]
	Artocarpus rigidus	Artonin F and cycloartobiloxanthonen	Multidrug-resistant (K1)	4.5 - 8.5	[108]
	Bauhinia purpurea	Demethoxymatteucinol	Multidrug-resistant (K1)	9.5	[109]
	Campnosperma panamensis	Lanaroflavone	CQ-resistant (W2)		[110]
	Dorstenia barteri	stipulin 4-Hydroxylonchocarpin and kanzonol B	CQ-resistant (W2)	2.2 - 5.1	[111]
	Erythrina fusca	Lonchocarpol A	Multi-drug-resistant (K1) and - sensitive (FCR3)	3.9	[112]
	Erythrina sacleuxii	5'-prenylpratensein, shinpterocarpin	CQ-sensitive (D6) and CQ-resistant (W2)	6.3	[113]
	Erythrina stricta	Erybraedin A, erystagallin A and 5-hydroxysophoranone	Multidrug resistant strain (K1)	5 - 9	[114]
	Erythrina subumbrans	Vogelin C and lespedezaflavanone B	Multidrug resistant strain (K1)	6.6 - 9.1	[114]
	Ochna integerrima	Novel biflavones	CQ-sensitive (FCR3) and CQ-resistant (K1)	0.08 - 5.2	[115]

(Table 1) contd.....

Class	Plant	Compound[*]	*P. falciparum* Strain Used	IC_{50} µM	Reference
	Piper hostmannianum	(–)-Methyllinderatin and linderatone	CQ-sensitive F32-Tanzania and CQ-resistant FcB1-Columbia strains	5.3 - 5.6	[116]
	Piptadenia pervillei	(+)-Cathechin 5-Gallate, (+)-catechin 3-gallate	CQ-resistant FcB1	1 - 1.2	[117]
	Wikstroemia indica	Sikokianin B and C	CQ-sensitive (FCR3) and CQ-resistant (K1)	4.5 - 7.1	[118]
Lignans	*Holostylis reniformis*	(7'R,8S,8'R)-4,5-dimethoxy-3',4'-methylenodioxy-2,7'-cyclolignan-7-one; (7'R,8S,8'R)-3',4,4',-tetramethoxy-2,7'-cyclolignan-7-one; (7'R,8R,8'S)-3',4,4',5-tetramethoxy-2,7'-cyclolignan-7-one; (7'R,8S,8'S)-3',4,4',5-tetramethoxy-2,7'-cyclolignan-7-one; (7'R,8S,8'S)-3',4'-dimethoxy-4,5-methylenodioxy-2,7'-cyclolignan-7-one	CQ-resistant isolate (BHz 26/86)	0.2 - 8[c]	[119]
	Rourea minor	Rourinoside	CQ-sensitive (D6) and CQ-resistant (W2)	2.1	[120]
Quinones	*Bauhinia purpurea*	Bauhinoxepin	Multidrug resistant strain (K1)	5.8	[119]
	Bulbine frutescens	Isoknipholone; sodium 4'-O-demethylknipholone 6'-O-sulfate	CQ-sensitive (D6) and CQ-resistant (W2)	0.28 - 7.9	[121]
	Harungana madagascariensis	Bazouanthrone, feruginin A, harunganin, harunganol A and B	CQ-resistant (W2)	1.8 - 5.0	[122]

(Table 1) contd.....

Class	Plant	Compound*	*P. falciparum* Strain Used	IC_{50} µM	Reference
	Kniphofia foliosa	10-(chrysophanol-7'-yl)-10-(□)-hydroxychrysophanol-9-anthrone and chryslandicin	CQ-sensitive (3D7)	0.5 - 1	[123]
	Psorospermum glaberrimum	Glaberianthrone; 3-geranyloxyemodin, anthrone, 3-prenyloxyemodin anthrone, 2-geranylemodin and bianthrone 1A	CQ-resistant (W2)	1.68 - 5.34	[124]
	Zhumeria majdae	12,16-dideoxy aegyptinone B	CQ-sensitive (D6) and CQ-resistant (W2)	4.4	[125]
Steroids	*Caralluma tuberculata*	12-O-benzoyl-20-O-acetyl 3β,12β,14β,20β-tetrahydroxy-(20S)-pregn-5-ene-6-deoxy-3-O-methyl-b-D-allopyranosyl(1-4)-β-D-cymaropyranosyl (1-4)-β-D-cymaropyranoside; 12-O-benzoyl-20-O-acetyl-3β, 7α,12β,14β,20β-tetrahydroxy-(20S)-pregn-5-ene-6-deoxy-3-O-methyl-β-D-allopyranosyl-(1-4)-β-D-cymaropyranosyl-(1,4)-b-D-cymaropyranoside	CQ-sensitive (D6) and CQ-resistant (W2)	6.5 - 7.4	[126]
Stilbenes	*Parthenocissus tricuspidata*	Piceid-(1-6)-b-D-glucopyranoside	CQ-sensitive (D10)	5.3	[127]
	Pleuropterus ciliinervis	(E)-resveratrol-3-O-a-L-rhamnopyranosyl-(1-2)-b-D-xylopyranoside	CQ-sensitive (D10)	3.9	[128]
Tannins	*Punica granatum*	ellagic acid, gallagic acid, punicalin and punicalagin	CQ-sensitive (D6) and CQ-resistant (W2)	7.5 - 8.8	[129]
Terpenoids					

(Table 1) contd.....

Class	Plant	Compound*	*P. falciparum* Strain Used	IC_{50} µM	Reference
Sesquiterpenes	*Anthemis auriculata*	4-Hydroxyanthecotulide	Enoyl-ACP reductase enzyme from P. falciparum	7.6	[130]
	Artemisia gorgonum	Hanphyllin	CQ-resistant (FcB1)	9.7	[131]
	Camchaya calcarea	Goyazensolide, lychnophorolide B, isogoyazensolide, isocentratherin, 5-epi-isogoyazensolide, 5-ep--isocentratherin	Multidrug resistant strain (K1)	3.3 - 8	[132]
	Cyperus articulatus	Corymbolone, mustakone	CQ-sensitive (NF 54), and CQ-resistant (ENT 36)	0.64 - 4.53	[133]
	Oncosiphon piluliferum	Sivasinolide, tavulin and tanachin	CQ-sensitive (D6) and CQ-resistant (W2)	1.5 - 9.8	[134]
	Vernonia cinerea	8 α -tigloyloxy-hirsutinolide-13-O-acetate, 8a-(4-hydroxyethacryloyloxy)-hirsutinolide-13-O-acetate, and vernolide D	CQ-resistant (W2)	3.5 - 3.9	[135]
	Vernonia staehelinoides	8α-(2-methylacryloyloxy)-3-oxo-1-desoxy-1,2-dehydrohirsutinolide-13-O-acetate, 8 α -(5--acetoxysenecioyloxy)-3-oxo-1-desoxy-1,2-dehydrohirsutinolide-13-O-acetate	CQ-sensitive (D10) and CQ-resistant (K1)	0.5 - 0.6	[136]
	Vernoniopsis caudate	Helenalin-[2-(1-hydroxyethyl)acrylate], helenalin-[2-hydroxyethyl-3-methyl)acrylate] and 11a,13-dihydrohelenalin-[2-(1-hydroxyethyl)acrylate]	CQ-resistant (FcB1)	0.19 - 1	[137]
	Wedelia trilobata Hitchc	Wedelolides A and B	Not indicated	4.2 - 9.1	[138]
Diterpenes					

(Table 1) contd.....

Class	Plant	Compound*	*P. falciparum* Strain Used	IC_{50} μM	Reference
	Aframomum zambesiacum	3-deoxyaulacocarpin A	CQ-resistant FCB1	4.97	[139]
	Caesalpinia bonduc	Bonducellpins	Multidrug-resistant (K1)	1.6 - 5.8	[140]
	Caesalpinia crista, Caesalpinia crista	Caesalpinins, norcaesalpinins, caesalmins	CQ-resistant (FCR-3/A2)	0.09 - 6.4	[141]
	Casearia grewiifolia	Caseargrewiins A–D	Multidrug-resistant (K1)	3.6 - 7.9	[142]
	Croton lobatus	Geranylgeraniol	Multidrug-resistant (K1)	3.7	[143]
	Croton steenkampianus	Steenkrotin A	CQ sensitive (D10 and D6) and CQ-resistant (Dd2 and W2)	9.1	[144]
	Juniperus seravschanica	Cedrol, sugiol, 12,15-dihydroxylabda-8(17),13-dien-19-oic acid	Multidrug-resistant (K1)	1.4 - 4.6	[145]
	Laetia procera	Casearlucin A, casamembrol A, laetiaprocerine A–D	CQ-sensitive (F32), CQ-resistant (FCb1)	0.5 - 6	[146]
	Simaba orinocensis	Orinocinolide, simalikalactone	CQ-sensitive (D6) and CQ-resistant (W2)	0.007 - 0.018	[147]

(Table 1) contd.....

Class	Plant	Compound*	*P. falciparum* Strain Used	IC_{50} μM	Reference
Triterpenes	*Chisocheton siamensis*	Dysobinin, mahonin	Multidrug-resistant (K1)	4.2 - 5.7	[148]
	Cogniauxia podolaena	Cucurbitacin B, cucurbitacin D, 20-epibryonolic acid	CQ-resistant (FcM29)	2.9 - 7.8	[149]
	Diospyros quaesita	Betulinic acid 3-caffeate	CQ-sensitive (D6) and CQ-resistant (W2)	0.98	[150]
	Ekebergia capensis	2,3,22,23-Tetrahydroxy-2,6,10,15,19,23-hexamethyl-6,10,14,18-tetracosatetraene (3R,22R)	CQ-sensitive (D6) and CQ-resistant (W2)	7	[151]
	Entandrophragma angolense	7α-obacunyl cetate	CQ-resistant (W2)	4	[152]
	Erythrina subumbrans; E. stricta	Soyasapogenol B	Multidrug-resistant (K1)	10	[153]
	Garcinia polyantha	Garcinane	Isolate NF54	2.5 - 4.1	[154]
	Grewia bilamellata	2α,3β-dihydroxyolean-12-en-28-oic acid	CQ-sensitive (D6) and CQ-resistant (W2)	8.6	[155]
	Harungana madagascariensis	Friedelan-3-one	CQ-resistant (W2)	7.7	[122]
	Khaya anthotheca	Anthothecol	CQ-resistant (W2)	0.17	[156]

(Table 1) contd.....

Class	Plant	Compound*	*P. falciparum* Strain Used	IC_{50} µM	Reference
	Lansium domesticum	Domesticulide B and C, methyl 6-acetoxyangolensate, azadiradione, dukunolide C	CQ-resistant (W2)	4.1 - 9.6	[157]
	Morinda lucida	Ursolic acid	CQ-sensitive (D6) and Multidrug-resistant (K1)	6.8	[158]
	Nauclea orientalis	3α,23-dihydroxyurs-12-en-28-oic acid	CQ-sensitive (D6)	9.7	[92]
	Nuxia sphaerocephala	3-oxolupenal, 3β-hydroxy-lupenal	CQ-resistant (FcB1)	3.6 - 7.2	[159]
	Picrolemma sprucei	Neosergeolide	Multidrug-resistant (K1)	2	[160]
	Pseudocedrela kotschyi	7-deacetylgedunin, 7-deacetyl-7-oxogedunin	Multidrug-resistant K1	3.1 - 4.1	[161]
	Salacia madagascariensis	20-epi-isoiguesterinol, isoiguesterin	CQ-sensitive (D6) and CQ-resistant (W2)	0.16 - 0.5	[162]
	Ziziphus cambodianus	3-O-vanillylceanothic acid, 2-O-E-p-coumaroyl alphitolic acid, zizyberenalic acid	Multidrug-resistant (K1)	1.5 - 6.6	[163]
Xanthones	*Allanblackia monticola*	Allanxanthone C, Tovophyllin, norcowanin, mangostin	CQ-sensitive (F32) and CQ-resistant (FcM29)	0.7 - 7.8	[164]
	Cratoxylum cochinchinense	5-O-methylcelebixanthone,	Multidrug-resistant (K1)	8.9	[165]
	Garcinia polyantha	Garciniaxanthon, smeathxanthone A, smeathxanthone B and chefouxanthone	Isolate NF54	2.5 - 4.1	[154]

(Table 1) contd.....

Class	Plant	Compound*	*P. falciparum* Strain Used	IC_{50} µM	Reference
	Swertia alata	Swertiaperennine, swertianin and decussatin,	*P. berghei*	5	[166]
	Symphonia globulifera	Gaboxanthone	CQ-resistant (W2	3.5	[167]
Others	*Cannabis sativa*	Cannabichromanone	CQ-sensitive (D6) and QC-resistant (W2)	9.4	[168]
	Cassia siamea	Chrobisiamone A	CQ-sensitive (3D7)	5.6	[169]
	Cussonia zimmermannii	8-hydroxyheptadeca-1-ene-4,6-diyn-3-yl ethanoate, 16-acetoxy-11-hydroxyoctadeca-17-ene-12,14-diynylethanoate	CQ-sensitive (D6)	1.4 - 2.2	[170]
	Garcinia polyantha	Isoxanthochymol	Isolate NF54	2.2	[154]
	Guiera senegalensis	Guieranone	CQ-resistant (W2)	4.1	[171]
	Machaerium multiflorum	Machaeriol A and B	CQ-sensitive (D6) and CQ-resistant (W2)	0.34 - 4.9	[172]
	Piper tricuspe	Dictyochromenol; 2'E,6'E 2-farnesyl hydroquinone	CQ-resistant (FcB1)	1.37 - 9.58	[173]
	Pothomorphe peltata	4-Nerolidylcatechol	Multidrug-resistant (K1)	0.67	[160]

(Table 1) contd.....

Class	Plant	Compound*	*P. falciparum* Strain Used	IC_{50} µM	Reference
	Rourea minor	Rouremin, 1-(26-hydroxyhexacosanoyl)-glycerol	CQ-sensitive (D6)	5.1 - 9.5	[92]
	Scrophularia cryptophilla	Crypthophilic acid C	Multidrug-resistant (K1)	4.1	[174]
	Symphonia globulifera	Guttiferone A	CQ-resistant (W2)	3.2	[167]

*Structures of compounds are readily accessible in the literatures (viz., SciFinder Scholar, Google Scholar, PubMed and CAS database). Up to [a]72%, [b]56%, [c]89%, [d]67% suppression of parasitemia in *P. berghei*-infected rodents.

CONCLUSION

Significant success has been historically recorded in antimalarial drug discovery from plants as typified by quinine, artemisinin and their several analogs. The discovery of the artemisinin has remained the strongest motivation for plant-based antimalarial drug research. In fact, Dr. Youyou Tu, one of the recipients of the 2015 Nobel Prize in Medicine, was awarded for her role in the discovery of artemisinin. This dominant role of natural products in antimalarial drug discovery has continued with appreciable success.

Reports of emerging resistance to existing antimalarial drugs have again necessitated a continuous search for effective alternatives and replacements. The overview of the recent advances provided in this chapter in this regards has highlighted the many studies on potential plant-derived antimalarial drugs. It presents the vast potential of herbal products to provide leads in antimalarial drug discovery. Importantly, several compounds that have shown potent antiplasmodial activity are highlighted providing insights into the existing gaps between basic and clinical antimalarial drug discovery. This update is hoped to provide guidance in research choices and policy decision towards antimalarial drugs discovery efforts.

CONFLICT OF INTEREST

The authors confirm that they have no conflict of interest to declare for this publication.

ACKNOWLEDGEMENTS

This work was supported by United States Agency for International Development (USAID) grant for Africa-U.S. Higher Education Partnership program [USAID/HED] Grant No HED153-6200-BFA-15-01 and USDA-ARS specific cooperative agreement No. 586408-1-603.

GLOSSARY

Alkaloids = Group of naturally occurring and organic nitrogen-containing bases with diverse physiological activity in humans and animals.

Anti-malarial drugs = Drugs/medicines and their products developed to prevent and treat malarial infections.

Artemisinin = Also known as qinghaosu, and its semi-synthetic derivatives are a group of drugs that possess the most rapid action of all current drugs against *Plasmodium falciparum* malaria.

Atovaquone = Chemical compound that belongs to the class of naphthoquinones. Atovaquone is a hydroxy-1,4-naphthoquinone, an analog of ubiquinone, with antipneumocystic and antimalarial activity.

Chloroquine = A 4-aminoquinoline compound use in the treatment and suppression of malaria cause by *Plasmodium vivax* , *P. malariae*, and *P. falciparum*. It is also used for hepatic amebiasis and for certain skin diseases including lupus erythematosus and lichen planus.

Cinchona = A genus of tree or shrub in the family Rubiaceae containing at least 23. Its dried bark is a source of quinine and other medicinal alkaloids.

Coumarins = Benzopyrone products that occur naturally in some plants. Some coumarins have been found to have medicinal uses. Others are used as precursor compounds to synthesize physiologically-active derivatives.

Drug discovery = A multi-disciplinary process through which new drugs and therapeutic agents are discovered and developed for the prevention and treatment of diseases.

Endoperoxides = Group of compounds whose chemical structures contain the peroxide moiety (-O-O-) as part of the larger structure.

Febrifugine = A quinazoline-type alkaloid which is the active principle in the Chinese antimalarial plant *Dichroa febrifuga* (Saxifragaceae), known locally as Ch'ang shan.

Flavonoids = Group of plant-derived compounds known for their anti-oxidant properties. Their general chemical structure consists of a 15-carbon skeleton, which consists of two phenyl rings and a heterocyclic ring.

Herbal medicine = Also referred to as phytomedicine, herbalism or botanical medicine, is the study or practice of using plants (whole or part) for medicinal purposes.

Lignans = Group of polyphenolic chemical compounds found in plants. Some isolated lignans have shown promising medicinal properties.

Malaria = An infectious disease caused by protozoan parasites from the Plasmodium family. The parasite can be transmitted through the bite of the Anopheles mosquito, contaminated needle or infected blood transfusion.

Parasitemia = The status of having parasites in the circulating blood. In malaria, the presence of Plasmodium in blood is often accompanied by fever and related symptoms. Asymptomatic parasitaemia' is a term used if no fever or other symptoms are present.

Plasmodium = Malaria parasites belonging to the phylum Apicomplexa. Most common species include *falciparum, malariae* and *vivax*.

Protozoan = Single-celled eukaryotic organisms which belong to the Kingdom Protista. While some protozoa are free-living, others including the malaria parasites are parasitic.

Quinine = An antimalarial compound isolated from cinchona bark.

Steroids = Class of organic compounds with a characteristic molecular structure containing four rings of carbon atoms (three six-membered and one five). They include many hormones and vitamins.

Structure-activity relationship = Relationship between the chemical structure of a compound and its biological activity. In drug discovery, particular attention is paid to the changes in biological activity of a compound occasioned by structural modification.

REFERENCES

[1] World Health Organization. Fact sheet on the World Malaria Report. 2014.

[2] Petersen I, Eastman R, Lanzer M. Drug-resistant malaria: molecular mechanisms and implications for public health. FEBS Lett 2011; 585(11): 1551-62.
[http://dx.doi.org/10.1016/j.febslet.2011.04.042] [PMID: 21530510]

[3] World Health Organization. Guidelines for the treatment of malaria. Geneva 2006.

[4] Dondorp AM, Nosten F, Yi P, *et al.* Artemisinin resistance in Plasmodium falciparum malaria. N Engl J Med 2009; 361(5): 455-67.
[http://dx.doi.org/10.1056/NEJMoa0808859] [PMID: 19641202]

[5] Djimde AA, Makanga M, Kuhen K, Hamed K. The emerging threat of artemisinin resistance in malaria: focus on artemether-lumefantrine. Expert Rev Anti Infect Ther 2015; 13(8): 1031-45.
[http://dx.doi.org/10.1586/14787210.2015.1052793] [PMID: 26081265]

[6] Nosten F, Brasseur P. Combination therapy for malaria: the way forward? Drugs 2002; 62(9): 1315-29.
[http://dx.doi.org/10.2165/00003495-200262090-00003] [PMID: 12076181]

[7] Kouznetsov VV, Gómez-Barrio A. Recent developments in the design and synthesis of hybrid molecules based on aminoquinoline ring and their antiplasmodial evaluation. Eur J Med Chem 2009; 44(8): 3091-113.
[http://dx.doi.org/10.1016/j.ejmech.2009.02.024] [PMID: 19361896]

[8] Soh PN, Benoit-Vical F. Are West African plants a source of future antimalarial drugs? J Ethnopharmacol 2007; 114(2): 130-40.
[http://dx.doi.org/10.1016/j.jep.2007.08.012] [PMID: 17884314]

[9] Jantz SM, Barker B, Brooks TM, *et al.* Future habitat loss and extinctions driven by land-use change in biodiversity hotspots under four scenarios of climate-change mitigation. Conserv Biol 2015; 29(4): 1122-31.
[http://dx.doi.org/10.1111/cobi.12549] [PMID: 26129841]

[10] Staba EJ, Chung AC. Quinine and quinidine production by cinchona leaf, root and unorganized cultures. Phytochemistry 1981; 20(11): 2495-8.
[http://dx.doi.org/10.1016/0031-9422(81)83079-8]

[11] Wells TN. Natural products as starting points for future anti-malarial therapies: going back to our roots? Malar J 2011; 10 (Suppl. 1): S3.
[http://dx.doi.org/10.1186/1475-2875-10-S1-S3] [PMID: 21411014]

[12] Tu Y. The discovery of artemisinin (qinghaosu) and gifts from Chinese medicine. Nat Med 2011; 17(10): 1217-20.
[http://dx.doi.org/10.1038/nm.2471] [PMID: 21989013]

[13] Trager W, Jensen JB. Human malaria parasites in continuous culture. Science 1976; 193(4254): 673-5.
[http://dx.doi.org/10.1126/science.781840] [PMID: 781840]

[14] Desjardins RE, Canfield CJ, Haynes JD, Chulay JD. Quantitative assessment of antimalarial activity *in vitro* by a semiautomated microdilution technique. Antimicrob Agents Chemother 1979; 16(6): 710-8.
[http://dx.doi.org/10.1128/AAC.16.6.710] [PMID: 394674]

[15] Makler MT, Ries JM, Williams JA, *et al.* Parasite lactate dehydrogenase as an assay for *Plasmodium falciparum* drug sensitivity. Am J Trop Med Hyg 1993; 48(6): 739-41.
[PMID: 8333566]

[16] Mazier M, Franetich M, Carraz M, Silvie O, Pino P. Models for studying the effects of herbal antimalarials at different stages of the *Plasmodium* life cycle. In: Willox M, Bodeker G, Rasoanaivo P, Eds. Traditional Medicinal Plants and Malaria. Boca Raton: CRC Press 2004; pp. 271-8.

[17] Bolscher JM, Koolen KM, van Gemert GJ, *et al.* A combination of new screening assays for prioritization of transmission-blocking antimalarials reveals distinct dynamics of marketed and experimental drugs. J Antimicrob Chemother 2015; 70(5): 1357-66.
[http://dx.doi.org/10.1093/jac/dkv003] [PMID: 25667405]

[18] Patwardhan B, Vaidya AD. Natural products drug discovery: accelerating the clinical candidate development using reverse pharmacology approaches. Indian J Exp Biol 2010; 48(3): 220-7.
[PMID: 21046974]

[19] Tu Y, Jeffries C, Ruan H, *et al.* Automated high-throughput system to fractionate plant natural products for drug discovery. J Nat Prod 2010; 73(4): 751-4.
[http://dx.doi.org/10.1021/np9007359] [PMID: 20232897]

[20] Yakoub AdenAbdi OE. Handbook of Drugs for Tropical Parasitic Infections. 1995.

[21] World Health Organization. Malaria treatment guidelines. 2010.

[22] Renslo AR. Antimalarial drug discovery: from quinine to the dream of eradication. ACS Med Chem Lett 2013; 4(12): 1126-8.
[http://dx.doi.org/10.1021/ml4004414] [PMID: 24790706]

[23] Rosenthal PJ. Antimalarial drug discovery: old and new approaches. J Exp Biol 2003; 206(Pt 21): 3735-44.
[http://dx.doi.org/10.1242/jeb.00589] [PMID: 14506208]

[24] Paterno E. On lapachic acid and its derivatives. J Franklin Inst 1889; 128(2): 139-40.
[http://dx.doi.org/10.1016/0016-0032(89)90170-1]

[25] Carvalho LH, Rocha EM, Raslan DS, Oliveira AB, Krettli AU. *In vitro* activity of natural and synthetic naphthoquinones against erythrocytic stages of Plasmodium falciparum. Braz J Med Biol Res 1988; 21(3): 485-7.
[PMID: 3067810]

[26] Fieser LF, Fawaz G. Naphthoquinone Antimalarials. XXIV. A New Synthesis of Lapinone. J Am

Chem Soc 1950; 72: 996-1000.
[http://dx.doi.org/10.1021/ja01158a091]

[27] Sherman IW. The road to atovaquone. Adv Parasitol 2008; 67: 101-4.
[http://dx.doi.org/10.1016/S0065-308X(08)00412-0]

[28] Posner GH, Parker MH, Northrop J, *et al.* Orally active, hydrolytically stable, semisynthetic, antimalarial trioxanes in the artemisinin family. J Med Chem 1999; 42(2): 300-4.
[http://dx.doi.org/10.1021/jm980529v] [PMID: 9925735]

[29] O'Neill PM, Searle NL, Kan KW, *et al.* Novel, potent, semisynthetic antimalarial carba analogues of the first-generation 1,2,4-trioxane artemether. J Med Chem 1999; 42(26): 5487-93.
[http://dx.doi.org/10.1021/jm9903545] [PMID: 10639291]

[30] Ma J, Weiss E, Kyle DE, Ziffer H. Acid catalyzed Michael additions to artemisitene. Bioorg Med Chem Lett 2000; 10(14): 1601-3.
[http://dx.doi.org/10.1016/S0960-894X(00)00297-3] [PMID: 10915061]

[31] Jefford CW, McGoran EC, Boukouvalas J, Richardson G, Robinson BL, Peters W. Synthesis of new 1,2,4-trioxanes and their antimalarial activity. Helv Chim Acta 1988; 1805-12.
[http://dx.doi.org/10.1002/hlca.19880710722]

[32] Kepler JA, Philip A, Lee YW, Musallam HA, Carroll FI. Endoperoxides as potential antimalarial agents. J Med Chem 1987; 30(8): 1505-9.
[http://dx.doi.org/10.1021/jm00391a039] [PMID: 3302259]

[33] Peters W, Robinson BL, Rossier JC, Jefford CW. The chemotherapy of rodent malaria. XLVIII. The activities of some synthetic 1,2,4-trioxanes against chloroquine-sensitive and chloroquine-resistant parasites. Part 1: Studies leading to the development of novel cis-fused cyclopenteno derivatives. Ann Trop Med Parasitol 1993; 87(1): 1-7.
[PMID: 8346987]

[34] Peters W, Robinson BL, Rossier JC, Misra D, Jefford CW, Rossiter JC. The chemotherapy of rodent malaria. XLIX. The activities of some synthetic 1,2,4-trioxanes against chloroquine-sensitive and chloroquine-resistant parasites. Part 2: Structure-activity studies on cis-fused cyclopenteno-1,2,--trioxanes (fenozans) against drug-sensitive and drug-resistant lines of Plasmodium berghei and P. yoelii ssp. NS *in vivo.* Ann Trop Med Parasitol 1993; 87(1): 9-16.
[PMID: 8346994]

[35] Vennerstrom JL, Dong Y, Andersen SL, *et al.* Synthesis and antimalarial activity of sixteen dispiro-1,2,4, 5-tetraoxanes: alkyl-substituted 7,8,15,16-tetraoxadispiro[5.2.5. 2]hexadecanes. J Med Chem 2000; 43(14): 2753-8.
[http://dx.doi.org/10.1021/jm0000766] [PMID: 10893313]

[36] Posner GH, Jeon HB, Parker MH, Krasavin M, Paik IH, Shapiro TA. Antimalarial simplified 3-aryltrioxanes: synthesis and preclinical efficacy/toxicity testing in rodents. J Med Chem 2001; 44(19): 3054-8.
[http://dx.doi.org/10.1021/jm0102396] [PMID: 11543673]

[37] Posner GH, Cumming JN, Woo SH, Ploypradith P, Xie S, Shapiro TA. Orally active antimalarial 3-substituted trioxanes: new synthetic methodology and biological evaluation. J Med Chem 1998; 41(6): 940-51.

[http://dx.doi.org/10.1021/jm970686e] [PMID: 9526568]

[38] Vennerstrom JL, Arbe-Barnes S, Brun R, *et al.* Identification of an antimalarial synthetic trioxolane drug development candidate. Nature 2004; 430(7002): 900-4. [http://dx.doi.org/10.1038/nature02779] [PMID: 15318224]

[39] Xu XX, Zhu J, Huang DZ, Zhou WS. Total synthesis of. Yingzhaosu A Tetrahedron Lett 1991; 32(41): 5785-8. [http://dx.doi.org/10.1016/S0040-4039(00)93555-X]

[40] Girometta MA, Jauch R, Ponelle C, Guenzi A, Wiegand-Chou RC. Animal pharmacokinetics and metabolism of the new antimalarial Ro 42-1611 (arteflene). Trop Med Parasitol 1994; 45(3): 272-7. [PMID: 7899803]

[41] Weidekamm E, Dumont E, Jaquet C. Tolerability and pharmacokinetics of Ro 42-1611 (arteflene) in man. Trop Med Parasitol 1994; 45(3): 278-83. [PMID: 7899804]

[42] Somo-Moyou R, Mittelholzer ML, Sorenson F, Haller L, Stürchler D. Efficacy of Ro 42-1611 (arteflene) in the treatment of patients with mild malaria: a clinical trial in Cameroon. Trop Med Parasitol 1994; 45(3): 288-91. [PMID: 7899806]

[43] Radloff PD, Philipps J, Nkeyi M, Sturchler D, Mittelholzer ML, Kremsner PG. Arteflene compared with mefloquine for treating Plasmodium falciparum malaria in children. Am J Trop Med Hyg 1996; 55(3): 259-62. [PMID: 8842111]

[44] Gellert E, Raymond-Hamet Schlittler E. The use of the plant Cryptolepis sanguinolenfa in folklore medicine. Helv Chim Acta 1951; 34: 642.

[45] Grellier P, Ramiaramanana L, Milleriox V, Deharo E, Shrevel J, Frappier F. Antimalarial activity of cryptolepine and isocryptolepine, alkaloids isolated from *Cryptolepis sanguinolenta.* Phytother Res 1996; 10: 317-21. [http://dx.doi.org/10.1002/(SICI)1099-1573(199606)10:4<317::AID-PTR858>3.0.CO;2-0]

[46] Wright CW, Phillipson JD, Awe SO, *et al.* Antimalarial activity of cryptolepine and some other anhydronium bases. Phytother Res 1996; 10: 361-3. [http://dx.doi.org/10.1002/(SICI)1099-1573(199606)10:4<361::AID-PTR845>3.0.CO;2-N]

[47] Cimanga K, De Bruyne T, Pieters L, Vlietinck AJ, Turger CA. *In vitro* and *in vivo* antiplasmodial activity of cryptolepine and related alkaloids from *Cryptolepis sanguinolenta.* J Nat Prod 1997; 60(7): 688-91. [http://dx.doi.org/10.1021/np9605246] [PMID: 9249972]

[48] Noamesi BK, Paine A, Kirby GC, Warhurst DC, Phillipson JD. *In vitro* antimalarial activity of cryptolepine, an indoquinoline. Trans R Soc Trop Med Hyg 1991; 85: 315.

[49] Kirby GC, Paine A, Warhurst DC, Noamesi BK, Phillipson JD. *In vitro* and *in vivo* antimalarial activity of cryptolepine, a plant-derived indoloquinoline. Phytother Res 1995; 9: 359-63. [http://dx.doi.org/10.1002/ptr.2650090510]

[50] Bugyei KA, Boye GL, Addy ME. Clinical efficacy of a tea-bag formulation of *Cryptolepis*

sanguinolenta root in the treatment of acute uncomplicated falciparum malaria. Ghana Med J 2010; 44(1): 3-9.
[PMID: 21326984]

[51] Lavrado J, Cabal GG, Prudêncio M, *et al.* Incorporation of basic side chains into cryptolepine scaffold: structure-antimalarial activity relationships and mechanistic studies. J Med Chem 2011; 54(3): 734-50.
[http://dx.doi.org/10.1021/jm101383f] [PMID: 21207937]

[52] Lavrado J, Paulo A, Gut J, Rosenthal PJ, Moreira R. Cryptolepine analogues containing basic aminoalkyl side-chains at C-11: synthesis, antiplasmodial activity, and cytotoxicity. Bioorg Med Chem Lett 2008; 18(4): 1378-81.
[http://dx.doi.org/10.1016/j.bmcl.2008.01.015] [PMID: 18207399]

[53] Mesia K, Cimanga RK, Dhooghe L, *et al.* Antimalarial activity and toxicity evaluation of a quantified *Nauclea pobeguinii* extract. J Ethnopharmacol 2010; 131(1): 10-6.
[http://dx.doi.org/10.1016/j.jep.2010.05.008] [PMID: 20470876]

[54] Mesia K, Cimanga K, Tona L, *et al.* Assessment of the short-term safety and tolerability of a quantified 80 % ethanol extract from the stem bark of *Nauclea pobeguinii* (PR 259 CT1) in healthy volunteers: a clinical phase I study. Planta Med 2011; 77(2): 111-6.
[http://dx.doi.org/10.1055/s-0030-1250134] [PMID: 20665369]

[55] Mesia K, Tona L, Mampunza MM, *et al.* Antimalarial efficacy of a quantified extract of *Nauclea pobeguinii* stem bark in human adult volunteers with diagnosed uncomplicated falciparum malaria. Part 1: a clinical phase IIA trial. Planta Med 2012; 78(3): 211-8.
[http://dx.doi.org/10.1055/s-0031-1280359] [PMID: 22095262]

[56] Mesia K, Tona L, Mampunza MM, *et al.* Antimalarial efficacy of a quantified extract of *Nauclea pobeguinii* stem bark in human adult volunteers with diagnosed uncomplicated falciparum malaria. Part 2: a clinical phase IIB trial. Planta Med 2012; 78(9): 853-60.
[http://dx.doi.org/10.1055/s-0031-1298488] [PMID: 22538476]

[57] Willcox ML, Graz B, Falquet J, Sidibé O, Forster M, Diallo D. Argemone mexicana decoction for the treatment of uncomplicated falciparum malaria. Trans R Soc Trop Med Hyg 2007; 101(12): 1190-8.
[http://dx.doi.org/10.1016/j.trstmh.2007.05.017] [PMID: 17920092]

[58] Graz B, Willcox ML, Diakite C, *et al. Argemone mexicana* decoction *versus* artesunate-amodiaquine for the management of malaria in Mali: policy and public-health implications. Trans R Soc Trop Med Hyg 2010; 104(1): 33-41.
[http://dx.doi.org/10.1016/j.trstmh.2009.07.005] [PMID: 19733875]

[59] Challand S. The use of medicinal plants in Kasese, Uganda. Trop Doct 2005; 35: 222-3.
[http://dx.doi.org/10.1258/004947505774938512] [PMID: 16354476]

[60] Hakizamungu E, Weri M. The use of medicinal plants in the treatment of malaria in Rwandan traditional medicine. Bull Med Trad Pharm 1988; 2: 11-7. [in French].

[61] Asase A, Oteng-Yeboah AA, Odamtten GT, Simmonds MS. Ethnobotanical study of some Ghanaian anti-malarial plants. J Ethnopharmacol 2005; 99(2): 273-9.
[http://dx.doi.org/10.1016/j.jep.2005.02.020] [PMID: 15894138]

[62] Ibrahim NG, Abdurahman EM, Ibrahim G. Elemental analysis of the leaves of *Vernonia amygdalina*

and its biological evaluation in rats. Niger J Nat Prod Med 2001; 5: 13-6.
[http://dx.doi.org/10.4314/njnpm.v5i1.11715]

[63] Iwalokun BA. Enhanced antimalarial effects of chloroquine by aqueous Vernonia amygdalina leaf extract in mice infected with chloroquine resistant and sensitive *Plasmodium berghei* strains. Afr Health Sci 2008; 8(1): 25-35.
[PMID: 19357729]

[64] Abosi AO, Raseroka BH. *In vivo* antimalarial activity of *Vernonia amygdalina.* Br J Biomed Sci 2003; 60(2): 89-91.
[PMID: 12866916]

[65] Erasto P, Grierson DS, Afolayan AJ. Bioactive sesquiterpene lactones from the leaves of *Vernonia amygdalina.* J Ethnopharmacol 2006; 106(1): 117-20.
[http://dx.doi.org/10.1016/j.jep.2005.12.016] [PMID: 16458461]

[66] Challand S, Willcox M. A clinical trial of *Veronia amygdalina* in the treatment of uncomplicated malaria. J Altern Complement Med 2009; 15: 1231-7.
[http://dx.doi.org/10.1089/acm.2009.0098] [PMID: 19922255]

[67] Jang CS, Fu FY, Huang KC, Wang CY. Pharmacology of ch'ang shan (Dichroa febrifuga) a Chinese antimalarial herb. Nature 1948; 161(4089): 400-1.
[http://dx.doi.org/10.1038/161400b0] [PMID: 18916817]

[68] Jang CS, Fu FY, Wang CY, Huang KC, Lu G, Chou TC. Ch'ang Shan, a Chinese Antimalarial Herb Science. Science 1946; 103: 59.
[http://dx.doi.org/10.1126/science.103.2663.59-b]

[69] Tang W, Eisenbrand G. Chinese Drugs of Plant Origin. Berlin, Germany: Springer-Verlag 1992; pp. 455-7.
[http://dx.doi.org/10.1007/978-3-642-73739-8_58]

[70] Kikuchi H, Yamamoto K, Horoiwa S, *et al.* Exploration of a new type of antimalarial compounds based on febrifugine. J Med Chem 2006; 49(15): 4698-706.
[http://dx.doi.org/10.1021/jm0601809] [PMID: 16854076]

[71] Kikuchi H, Horoiwa S, Kasahara R, Hariguchi N, Matsumoto M, Oshima Y. Synthesis of febrifugine derivatives and development of an effective and safe tetrahydroquinazoline-type antimalarial. Eur J Med Chem 2014; 76: 10-9.
[http://dx.doi.org/10.1016/j.ejmech.2014.01.036] [PMID: 24565569]

[72] Takaya Y, Tasaka H, Chiba T, *et al.* New type of febrifugine analogues, bearing a quinolizidine moiety, show potent antimalarial activity against Plasmodium malaria parasite. J Med Chem 1999; 42(16): 3163-6.
[http://dx.doi.org/10.1021/jm990131e] [PMID: 10447961]

[73] Sen D, Chatterjee TK. Pharmacophore modeling and 3D quantitative structure-activity relationship analysis of febrifugine analogues as potent antimalarial agent. J Adv Pharm Technol Res 2013; 4(1): 50-60.
[http://dx.doi.org/10.4103/2231-4040.107501] [PMID: 23662282]

[74] Daugschies A, Gässlein U, Rommel M. Comparative efficacy of anticoccidials under the conditions of

commercial broiler production and in battery trials. Vet Parasitol 1998; 76(3): 163-71. [http://dx.doi.org/10.1016/S0304-4017(97)00203-3] [PMID: 9615950]

[75] Peeters JE, Villacorta I, Naciri M, Vanopdenbosch E. Specific serum and local antibody responses against *Cryptosporidium parvum* during medication of calves with halofuginone lactate. Infect Immun 1993; 61(10): 4440-5. [PMID: 8406835]

[76] Jiang S, Zeng Q, Gettayacamin M, *et al.* Antimalarial activities and therapeutic properties of febrifugine analogs. Antimicrob Agents Chemother 2005; 49(3): 1169-76. [http://dx.doi.org/10.1128/AAC.49.3.1169-1176.2005] [PMID: 15728920]

[77] Geary TG, Divo AA, Jensen JB. Stage specific actions of antimalarial drugs on Plasmodium falciparum in culture. Am J Trop Med Hyg 1989; 40(3): 240-4. [PMID: 2648881]

[78] Derbyshire ER, Mazitschek R, Clardy J. Characterization of Plasmodium liver stage inhibition by halofuginone. ChemMedChem 2012; 7(5): 844-9. [http://dx.doi.org/10.1002/cmdc.201200045] [PMID: 22438279]

[79] Zhou H, Sun L, Yang XL, Schimmel P. ATP-directed capture of bioactive herbal-based medicine on human tRNA synthetase. Nature 2013; 494(7435): 121-4. [http://dx.doi.org/10.1038/nature11774] [PMID: 23263184]

[80] Caniato R, Puricelli L. Review: natural antimalarial agents (1995-2001). Crit Rev Plant Sci 2003; 22(1): 79-105. [http://dx.doi.org/10.1080/713610851]

[81] Bero J, Frédérich M, Quetin-Leclercq J. Antimalarial compounds isolated from plants used in traditional medicine. J Pharm Pharmacol 2009; 61(11): 1401-33. [http://dx.doi.org/10.1211/jpp.61.11.0001] [PMID: 19903367]

[82] Wright CW. Traditional antimalarials and the development of novel antimalarial drugs. J Ethnopharmacol 2005; 100(1-2): 67-71. [http://dx.doi.org/10.1016/j.jep.2005.05.012] [PMID: 16023812]

[83] Rukunga GM, Muregi FW, Tolo FM, *et al.* The antiplasmodial activity of spermine alkaloids isolated from *Albizia gummifera.* Fitoterapia 2007; 78(7-8): 455-9. [http://dx.doi.org/10.1016/j.fitote.2007.02.012] [PMID: 17601685]

[84] Samoylenko V, Jacob MR, Khan SI, *et al.* Antimicrobial, antiparasitic and cytotoxic spermine alkaloids from *Albizia schimperiana.* Nat Prod Commun 2009; 4(6): 791-6. [PMID: 19634324]

[85] Van Miert S, Hostyn S, Maes BU, *et al.* Isoneocryptolepine, a synthetic indoloquinoline alkaloid, as an antiplasmodial lead compound. J Nat Prod 2005; 68(5): 674-7. [http://dx.doi.org/10.1021/np0496284] [PMID: 15921407]

[86] Nguyen NT, Pham VC, Litaudon M, *et al.* Antiplasmodial alkaloids from Desmos rostrata. J Nat Prod 2008; 71(12): 2057-9. [http://dx.doi.org/10.1021/np8004437] [PMID: 19053513]

[87] Muhammad I, Dunbar DC, Takamatsu S, Walker LA, Clark AM. Antimalarial, cytotoxic, and

antifungal alkaloids from *Duguetia hadrantha.* J Nat Prod 2001; 64(5): 559-62. [http://dx.doi.org/10.1021/np000436s] [PMID: 11374943]

[88] Zirihi GN, Grellier P, Guédé-Guina F, Bodo B, Mambu L. Isolation, characterization and antiplasmodial activity of steroidal alkaloids from *Funtumia elastica* (Preuss) Stapf. Bioorg Med Chem Lett 2005; 15(10): 2637-40. [http://dx.doi.org/10.1016/j.bmcl.2005.03.021] [PMID: 15863333]

[89] Rumalla CS, Jadhav AN, Smillie T, Fronczek FR, Khan IA. Alkaloids from Heimia salicifolia. Phytochemistry 2008; 69(8): 1756-62. [http://dx.doi.org/10.1016/j.phytochem.2008.01.028] [PMID: 18374955]

[90] Toriizuka Y, *et al.* New lycorine-type alkaloid from Lycoris traubii and evaluation of antitrypanosomal and antimalarial activities of lycorine derivatives. Bioorg Med Chem 2008; 16: 10 182-9. [http://dx.doi.org/10.1016/j.bmc.2008.10.061]

[91] Phrutivorapongkul A, Ichino C, Ruangrungsi N. Anti-plasmodial activity of bisbenzylisoquinoline alkaloids from Michelia figo leaves. Thai J Health Res 2006; 20: 121-9.

[92] Sun J, Lou H, Dai S, Xu H, Zhao F, Liu K. Indole alkoloids from Nauclea officinalis with weak antimalarial activity. Phytochemistry 2008; 69(6): 1405-10. [http://dx.doi.org/10.1016/j.phytochem.2008.01.008] [PMID: 18328515]

[93] He ZD, Ma CY, Zhang HJ, *et al.* Antimalarial constituents from Nauclea orientalis (L.) L. Chem Biodivers 2005; 2(10): 1378-86. [http://dx.doi.org/10.1002/cbdv.200590110] [PMID: 17191939]

[94] Kanokmedhakul S, Kanokmedhakul K, Lekphrom R. Bioactive constituents of the roots of Polyalthia cerasoides. J Nat Prod 2007; 70(9): 1536-8. [http://dx.doi.org/10.1021/np070293a] [PMID: 17845001]

[95] Samoylenko V, Ashfaq MK, Jacob MR, *et al.* Indolizidine, antiinfective and antiparasitic compounds from Prosopis glandulosa var. glandulosa. J Nat Prod 2009; 72(1): 92-8. [http://dx.doi.org/10.1021/np800653z] [PMID: 19105653]

[96] Roumy V, Fabre N, Souard F, *et al.* Isolation and antimalarial activity of alkaloids from Pseudoxandra cuspidata. Planta Med 2006; 72(10): 894-8. [http://dx.doi.org/10.1055/s-2006-947184] [PMID: 16902855]

[97] Muhammad I, Dunbar DC, Khan SI, *et al.* Antiparasitic alkaloids from *Psychotria klugii.* J Nat Prod 2003; 66(7): 962-7. [http://dx.doi.org/10.1021/np030086k] [PMID: 12880315]

[98] Devkota KP, Lenta BN, Choudhary MI, *et al.* Cholinesterase inhibiting and antiplasmodial steroidal alkaloids from *Sarcococca hookeriana.* Chem Pharm Bull (Tokyo) 2007; 55(9): 1397-401. [http://dx.doi.org/10.1248/cpb.55.1397] [PMID: 17827771]

[99] Chea A, Hout S, Bun SS, *et al.* Antimalarial activity of alkaloids isolated from *Stephania rotunda.* J Ethnopharmacol 2007; 112(1): 132-7. [http://dx.doi.org/10.1016/j.jep.2007.02.005] [PMID: 17382502]

[100] Jullian V, Bourdy G, Georges S, Maurel S, Sauvain M. Validation of use of a traditional antimalarial remedy from French Guiana, *Zanthoxylum rhoifolium Lam.* J Ethnopharmacol 2006; 106(3): 348-52.

[http://dx.doi.org/10.1016/j.jep.2006.01.011] [PMID: 16504432]

[101] Murebwayire S, Frédérich M, Hannaert V, Jonville MC, Duez P. Antiplasmodial and antitrypanosomal activity of *Triclisia sacleuxii* (Pierre) Diels. Phytomedicine 2008; 15(9): 728-33. [http://dx.doi.org/10.1016/j.phymed.2007.10.005] [PMID: 18321694]

[102] Ross SA, Krishnaven K, Radwan MM, Takamatsu S, Burandt CL. Constituents of *Zanthoxylum flavum* and their antioxidant and antimalarial activities. Nat Prod Commun 2008; 3: 791-4.

[103] Ross SA, Al-Azeib MA, Krishnaveni KS, Fronczek FR, Burandt CL. Alkamides from the leaves of Zanthoxylum syncarpum. J Nat Prod 2005; 68(8): 1297-9. [http://dx.doi.org/10.1021/np0580558] [PMID: 16124784]

[104] Suksamrarn S, *et al.* Ziziphine N, O, P and Q, new antiplasmodial cyclopeptide alkaloids from *Ziziphus oenoplia* var. brunoniana. Tetrahedron 2005; 61: 1175-80. [http://dx.doi.org/10.1016/j.tet.2004.11.053]

[105] Subeki S, Matsuura H, Takahashi K, *et al.* Anti-babesial and anti-plasmodial compounds from Phyllanthus niruri. J Nat Prod 2005; 68(4): 537-9. [http://dx.doi.org/10.1021/np0497245] [PMID: 15844943]

[106] Boonphong S, Baramee A, Kittakoop P, Puangsombat P. Antitubercular and antiplasmodial prenylated flavones from the roots of *Artocarpus altilis*. Chiang Mai J Sci 2007; 34: 339-44.

[107] Widyawaruyanti A. New prenylated flavones from Artocarpus champeden, and their antimalarial activity *in vitro.* J Nat Med 2007; 61: 410-3. [http://dx.doi.org/10.1007/s11418-007-0153-8]

[108] Namdaung U, Aroonrerk N, Suksamrarn S, *et al.* Bioactive constituents of the root bark of *Artocarpus rigidus* subsp. rigidus. Chem Pharm Bull (Tokyo) 2006; 54(10): 1433-6. [http://dx.doi.org/10.1248/cpb.54.1433] [PMID: 17015984]

[109] Boonphong S, Puangsombat P, Baramee A, Mahidol C, Ruchirawat S, Kittakoop P. Bioactive compounds from *Bauhinia purpurea* possessing antimalarial, antimycobacterial, antifungal, anti-inflammatory, and cytotoxic activities. J Nat Prod 2007; 70(5): 795-801. [http://dx.doi.org/10.1021/np070010e] [PMID: 17480099]

[110] Weniger B, Vonthron-Sénécheau C, Arango GJ, Kaiser M, Brun R, Anton R. A bioactive biflavonoid from *Campnosperma panamense*. Fitoterapia 2004; 75(7-8): 764-7. [http://dx.doi.org/10.1016/j.fitote.2004.09.015] [PMID: 15567260]

[111] Ngameni B, Watchueng J, Boyom FF, *et al.* Antimalarial prenylated chalcones from the twigs of *Dorstenia barteri* var. subtriangularis. ARKIVOC 2007; xiii: 116-23.

[112] Khaomek P, Ichino C, Ishiyama A, *et al. In vitro* antimalarial activity of prenylated flavonoids from *Erythrina fusca*. J Nat Med 2008; 62(2): 217-20. [http://dx.doi.org/10.1007/s11418-007-0214-z] [PMID: 18404327]

[113] Andayi AW, Yenesew A, Derese S, *et al.* Antiplasmodial flavonoids from *Erythrina sacleuxii*. Planta Med 2006; 72(2): 187-9. [http://dx.doi.org/10.1055/s-2005-873200] [PMID: 16491458]

[114] Rukachaisirikul T, Saekee A, Tharibun C, Watkuolham S, Suksamrarn A. Biological activities of the chemical constituents of *Erythrina stricta* and *Erythrina subumbrans*. Arch Pharm Res 2007; 30(11):

1398-403.
[http://dx.doi.org/10.1007/BF02977363] [PMID: 18087807]

[115] Ichino C, Kiyohara H, Soonthornchareonnon N, *et al.* Antimalarial activity of biflavonoids from *Ochna integerrima*. Planta Med 2006; 72(7): 611-4.
[http://dx.doi.org/10.1055/s-2006-931569] [PMID: 16732520]

[116] Portet B, Fabre N, Roumy V, *et al.* Activity-guided isolation of antiplasmodial dihydrochalcones and flavanones from *Piper hostmannianum* var. berbicense. Phytochemistry 2007; 68(9): 1312-20.
[http://dx.doi.org/10.1016/j.phytochem.2007.02.006] [PMID: 17397884]

[117] Ramanandraibe V, Grellier P, Martin MT, *et al.* Antiplasmodial phenolic compounds from Piptadenia pervillei. Planta Med 2008; 74(4): 417-21.
[http://dx.doi.org/10.1055/s-2008-1034328] [PMID: 18484535]

[118] Nunome S, Ishiyama A, Kobayashi M, *et al. In vitro* antimalarial activity of biflavonoids from Wikstroemia indica. Planta Med 2004; 70(1): 76-8.
[http://dx.doi.org/10.1055/s-2004-815462] [PMID: 14765300]

[119] de Andrade-Neto VF, da Silva T, Lopes LM, do Rosário VE, de Pilla Varotti F, Krettli AU. Antiplasmodial activity of aryltetralone lignans from Holostylis reniformis. Antimicrob Agents Chemother 2007; 51(7): 2346-50.
[http://dx.doi.org/10.1128/AAC.01344-06] [PMID: 17438049]

[120] He ZD, Ma CY, Tan GT, *et al.* Rourinoside and rouremin, antimalarial constituents from Rourea minor. Phytochemistry 2006; 67(13): 1378-84.
[http://dx.doi.org/10.1016/j.phytochem.2006.04.012] [PMID: 16762381]

[121] Mutanyatta J, Bezabih M, Abegaz BM, *et al.* The first 6'-O-sulfated phenylanthraquinones: isolation from Bulbine frutescens, structural elucidation, enantiomeric purity, and partial synthesis. Tetrahedron 2005; 61: 8475-84.
[http://dx.doi.org/10.1016/j.tet.2005.06.055]

[122] Ndjakou Lenta B, Ngouela S, Fekam Boyom F, *et al.* Anti-plasmodial activity of some constituents of the root bark of *Harungana madagascariensis* LAM. (Hypericaceae). Chem Pharm Bull (Tokyo) 2007; 55(3): 464-7.
[http://dx.doi.org/10.1248/cpb.55.464] [PMID: 17329893]

[123] Wube AA, Bucar F, Asres K, Gibbons S, Rattray L, Croft SL. Antimalarial compounds from Kniphofia foliosa roots. Phytother Res 2005; 19(6): 472-6.
[http://dx.doi.org/10.1002/ptr.1635] [PMID: 16114082]

[124] Ndjakou Lenta B, Devkota KP, Ngouela S, *et al.* Anti-plasmodial and cholinesterase inhibiting activities of some constituents of *Psorospermum glaberrimum*. Chem Pharm Bull (Tokyo) 2008; 56(2): 222-6.
[http://dx.doi.org/10.1248/cpb.56.222] [PMID: 18239315]

[125] Moein MR, Pawar RS, Khan SI, Tekwani BL, Khan IA. Antileishmanial, antiplasmodial and cytotoxic activities of 12,16-dideoxy aegyptinone B from *Zhumeria majdae* Rech.f. & Wendelbo. Phytother Res 2008; 22(3): 283-5.
[http://dx.doi.org/10.1002/ptr.2305] [PMID: 17886231]

[126] Abdel-Sattar E, Harraz FM, Al-ansari SM, *et al.* Acylated pregnane glycosides from Caralluma tuberculata and their antiparasitic activity. Phytochemistry 2008; 69(11): 2180-6. [http://dx.doi.org/10.1016/j.phytochem.2008.05.017] [PMID: 18614190]

[127] Son IH, Chung IM, Lee SJ, Moon HI. Antiplasmodial activity of novel stilbene derivatives isolated from Parthenocissus tricuspidata from South Korea. Parasitol Res 2007; 101(1): 237-41. [http://dx.doi.org/10.1007/s00436-006-0454-y] [PMID: 17211658]

[128] Lee SI, Yang HD, Son IH, Moon HI. Antimalarial activity of a stilbene glycoside from *Pleuropterus ciliinervis*. Ann Trop Med Parasitol 2008; 102(2): 181-4. [http://dx.doi.org/10.1179/136485908X252359] [PMID: 18318941]

[129] Reddy MK, Gupta SK, Jacob MR, Khan SI, Ferreira D. Antioxidant, antimalarial and antimicrobial activities of tannin-rich fractions, ellagitannins and phenolic acids from *Punica granatum* L. Planta Med 2007; 73(5): 461-7. [http://dx.doi.org/10.1055/s-2007-967167] [PMID: 17566148]

[130] Karioti A, Skaltsa H, Zhang X, *et al.* Inhibiting enoyl-ACP reductase (FabI) across pathogenic microorganisms by linear sesquiterpene lactones from *Anthemis auriculata*. Phytomedicine 2008; 15(12): 1125-9. [http://dx.doi.org/10.1016/j.phymed.2008.02.018] [PMID: 18424102]

[131] Ortet R, Prado S, Mouray E, Thomas OP. Sesquiterpene lactones from the endemic Cape Verdean *Artemisia gorgonum*. Phytochemistry 2008; 69(17): 2961-5. [http://dx.doi.org/10.1016/j.phytochem.2008.09.022] [PMID: 19007951]

[132] Vongvanich N, Kittakoop P, Charoenchai P, Intamas S, Sriklung K, Thebtaranonth Y. Antiplasmodial, antimycobacterial, and cytotoxic principles from *Camchaya calcarea*. Planta Med 2006; 72(15): 1427-30. [http://dx.doi.org/10.1055/s-2006-951711] [PMID: 17089326]

[133] Rukunga GM, Muregi FW, Omar SA, *et al.* Anti-plasmodial activity of the extracts and two sesquiterpenes from *Cyperus articulatus*. Fitoterapia 2008; 79(3): 188-90. [http://dx.doi.org/10.1016/j.fitote.2007.11.010] [PMID: 18234452]

[134] Pillay P, Vleggaar R, Maharaj VJ, Smith PJ, Lategan CA. Isolation and identification of antiplasmodial sesquiterpene lactones from Oncosiphon piluliferum. J Ethnopharmacol 2007; 112(1): 71-6. [http://dx.doi.org/10.1016/j.jep.2007.02.002] [PMID: 17350777]

[135] Chea A, Hout S, Long C, *et al.* Antimalarial activity of sesquiterpene lactones from Vernonia cinerea. Chem Pharm Bull (Tokyo) 2006; 54(10): 1437-9. [http://dx.doi.org/10.1248/cpb.54.1437] [PMID: 17015985]

[136] Pillay P, Vleggaar R, Maharaj VJ, *et al.* Antiplasmodial hirsutinolides from Vernonia staehelinoides and their utilization towards a simplified pharmacophore. Phytochemistry 2007; 68(8): 1200-5. [http://dx.doi.org/10.1016/j.phytochem.2007.02.019] [PMID: 17408709]

[137] Ramanandraibe V, Martin MT, Rakotondramanana DL, *et al.* Pseudoguanolide sesquiterpene lactones from *Vernoniopsis caudata* and their *in vitro* antiplasmodial activities. J Nat Prod 2005; 68(5): 800-3. [http://dx.doi.org/10.1021/np0401866] [PMID: 15921436]

[138] That QT, Jossang J, Jossang A, Kim PP, Jaureguiberry G. Wedelolides A and B: novel sesquiterpene delta-lactones, (9R)-eudesman-9,12-olides, from *Wedelia trilobata.* J Org Chem 2007; 72(19): 7102-5. [http://dx.doi.org/10.1021/jo070771m] [PMID: 17705534]

[139] Kenmogne M, Prost E, Harakat D, *et al.* Five labdane diterpenoids from the seeds of *Aframomum zambesiacum*. Phytochemistry 2006; 67(5): 433-8. [http://dx.doi.org/10.1016/j.phytochem.2005.10.015] [PMID: 16321410]

[140] Pudhom K, Sommit D, Suwankitti N, Petsom A. Cassane furanoditerpenoids from the seed kernels of Caesalpinia bonduc from Thailand. J Nat Prod 2007; 70(9): 1542-4. [http://dx.doi.org/10.1021/np070330y] [PMID: 17848088]

[141] Linn TZ, Awale S, Tezuka Y, *et al.* Cassane- and norcassane-type diterpenes from Caesalpinia crista of Indonesia and their antimalarial activity against the growth of *Plasmodium falciparum*. J Nat Prod 2005; 68(5): 706-10. [http://dx.doi.org/10.1021/np0401720] [PMID: 15921414]

[142] Kanokmedhakul S, Kanokmedhakul K, Kanarsa T, Buayairaksa M. New bioactive clerodane diterpenoids from the bark of *Casearia grewiifolia*. J Nat Prod 2005; 68(2): 183-8. [http://dx.doi.org/10.1021/np049757k] [PMID: 15730240]

[143] Attioua B, Weniger B, Chabert P. Antiplasmodial activity of constituents isolated from Croton lobatus. Pharm Biol 2007; 45: 263-6. [http://dx.doi.org/10.1080/13880200701214607]

[144] Adelekan AM, Prozesky EA, Hussein AA, *et al.* Bioactive diterpenes and other constituents of *Croton steenkampianus*. J Nat Prod 2008; 71(11): 1919-22. [http://dx.doi.org/10.1021/np800333r] [PMID: 18855442]

[145] Okasaka M, Takaishi Y, Kashiwada Y, *et al.* Terpenoids from *Juniperus polycarpus* var. seravschanica. Phytochemistry 2006; 67(24): 2635-40. [http://dx.doi.org/10.1016/j.phytochem.2006.07.020] [PMID: 16956634]

[146] Jullian V, Bonduelle C, Valentin A, *et al.* New clerodane diterpenoids from Laetia procera (Poepp.) Eichler (Flacourtiaceae), with antiplasmodial and antileishmanial activities. Bioorg Med Chem Lett 2005; 15(22): 5065-70. [http://dx.doi.org/10.1016/j.bmcl.2005.07.090] [PMID: 16168652]

[147] Muhammad I, Bedir E, Khan SI, *et al.* A new antimalarial quassinoid from Simaba orinocensis. J Nat Prod 2004; 67(5): 772-7. [http://dx.doi.org/10.1021/np030524n] [PMID: 15165136]

[148] Maneerat W, Laphookhieo S, Koysomboon S, Chantrapromma K. Antimalarial, antimycobacterial and cytotoxic limonoids from *Chisocheton siamensis*. Phytomedicine 2008; 15(12): 1130-4. [http://dx.doi.org/10.1016/j.phymed.2008.05.004] [PMID: 18617378]

[149] Banzouzi JT, Soh PN, Mbatchi B, *et al.* Cogniauxia podolaena: bioassay-guided fractionation of defoliated stems, isolation of active compounds, antiplasmodial activity and cytotoxicity. Planta Med 2008; 74(12): 1453-6. [http://dx.doi.org/10.1055/s-2008-1081341] [PMID: 18704883]

[150] Ma CY, Musoke SF, Tan GT, *et al.* Study of antimalarial activity of chemical constituents from

Diospyros quaesita. Chem Biodivers 2008; 5(11): 2442-8.
[http://dx.doi.org/10.1002/cbdv.200890209] [PMID: 19035573]

[151] Murata T, Miyase T, Muregi FW, *et al.* Antiplasmodial triterpenoids from *Ekebergia capensis*. J Nat Prod 2008; 71(2): 167-74.
[http://dx.doi.org/10.1021/np0780093] [PMID: 18220356]

[152] Bickii J, Tchouya GR, Tchouankeu JC, Tsamo E. The antiplasmodial agents of the stem bark of *Entandrophragma angolense* (Meliaceae). Afr J Tradit Complement Altern Medicines 2006; 4(2): 135-9.
[PMID: 20162084]

[153] Rukachaisirikul T, Saekee A, Tharibun C, Watkuolham S, Suksamrarn A. Biological activities of the chemical constituents of *Erythrina stricta* and *Erythrina subumbrans*. Arch Pharm Res 2007; 30(11): 1398-403.
[http://dx.doi.org/10.1007/BF02977363] [PMID: 18087807]

[154] Lannang AM, Louh GN, Lontsi D, *et al.* Antimalarial compounds from the root bark of Garcinia polyantha Olv. J Antibiot 2008; 61(8): 518-23.
[http://dx.doi.org/10.1038/ja.2008.70] [PMID: 18997392]

[155] Ma C, Zhang HJ, Tan GT, *et al.* Antimalarial compounds from *Grewia bilamellata*. J Nat Prod 2006; 69(3): 346-50.
[http://dx.doi.org/10.1021/np050313d] [PMID: 16562832]

[156] Lee SE, Kim MR, Kim JH, Takeoka GR, Kim TW, Park BS. Antimalarial activity of anthothecol derived from Khaya anthotheca (Meliaceae). Phytomedicine 2008; 15(6-7): 533-5.
[http://dx.doi.org/10.1016/j.phymed.2007.08.001] [PMID: 17913482]

[157] Saewan N, Sutherland JD, Chantrapromma K. Antimalarial tetranortriterpenoids from the seeds of *Lansium domesticum* Corr. Phytochemistry 2006; 67(20): 2288-93.
[http://dx.doi.org/10.1016/j.phytochem.2006.07.005] [PMID: 16930641]

[158] Cimanga RK, Tona GL, Mesia GK, *et al.* Bioassay-guided isolation of antimalarial triterpenoid acids from the leaves of Morinda lucida. Pharm Biol 2006; 44: 677-81.
[http://dx.doi.org/10.1080/13880200601009123]

[159] Mambu L, Grellier P, Florent L, *et al.* Clerodane and labdane diterpenoids from Nuxia sphaerocephala. Phytochemistry 2006; 67(5): 444-51.
[http://dx.doi.org/10.1016/j.phytochem.2005.11.024] [PMID: 16427101]

[160] de Andrade-Neto VF, Pohlit AM, Pinto AC, *et al. In vitro* inhibition of *Plasmodium falciparum* by substances isolated from Amazonian antimalarial plants. Mem Inst Oswaldo Cruz 2007; 102(3): 359-65.
[PMID: 17568942]

[161] Hay AE, Ioset JR, Ahua KM, Diallo D, Brun R, Hostettmann K. Limonoid orthoacetates and antiprotozoal compounds from the roots of *Pseudocedrela kotschyi*. J Nat Prod 2007; 70(1): 9-13.
[http://dx.doi.org/10.1021/np0680230] [PMID: 17253841]

[162] Thiem DA, Sneden AT, Khan SI, Tekwani BL. Bisnortriterpenes from Salacia madagascariensis. J Nat Prod 2005; 68(2): 251-4.

[http://dx.doi.org/10.1021/np0497088] [PMID: 15730255]

[163] Suksamrarn S, Panseeta P, Kunchanawatta S, Distaporn T, Ruktasing S, Suksamrarn A. Ceanothane- and lupane-type triterpenes with antiplasmodial and antimycobacterial activities from Ziziphus cambodiana. Chem Pharm Bull (Tokyo) 2006; 54(4): 535-7. [http://dx.doi.org/10.1248/cpb.54.535] [PMID: 16595959]

[164] Azebaze AG, Meyer M, Valentin A, Nguemfo EL, Fomum ZT, Nkengfack AE. Prenylated xanthone derivatives with antiplasmodial activity from Allanblackia monticola STANER L.C. Chem Pharm Bull (Tokyo) 2006; 54(1): 111-3. [http://dx.doi.org/10.1248/cpb.54.111] [PMID: 16394561]

[165] Laphookhieo S, Syers JK, Kiattansakul R, Chantrapromma K. Cytotoxic and antimalarial prenylated xanthones from *Cratoxylum cochinchinense*. Chem Pharm Bull (Tokyo) 2006; 54(5): 745-7. [http://dx.doi.org/10.1248/cpb.54.745] [PMID: 16651783]

[166] Karan M, Bhatnagar S, Wangtak P, Vasisht K. Phytochemical and antimalarial studies on Swertia alata Royale. Acta Hortic 2005; 675: 139-45. [http://dx.doi.org/10.17660/ActaHortic.2005.675.20]

[167] Ngouela S, Lenta BN, Noungoue DT, *et al.* Anti-plasmodial and antioxidant activities of constituents of the seed shells of *Symphonia globulifera* Linn f. Phytochemistry 2006; 67(3): 302-6. [http://dx.doi.org/10.1016/j.phytochem.2005.11.004] [PMID: 16368120]

[168] Ahmed SA, Ross SA, Slade D, Radwan MM, Khan IA, Elsohly MA. Structure determination and absolute configuration of cannabichromanone derivatives from high potency *Cannabis sativa*. Tetrahedron Lett 2008; 49(42): 6050-3. [http://dx.doi.org/10.1016/j.tetlet.2008.07.178] [PMID: 19844597]

[169] Oshimi S, Tomizawa Y, Hirasawa Y, *et al.* Chrobisiamone A, a new bischromone from Cassia siamea and a biomimetic transformation of 5-acetonyl-7-hydroxy-2-methylchromone into cassiarin A. Bioorg Med Chem Lett 2008; 18(13): 3761-3. [http://dx.doi.org/10.1016/j.bmcl.2008.05.041] [PMID: 18524594]

[170] Senn M, Gunzenhauser S, Brun R, Séquin U. Antiprotozoal polyacetylenes from the Tanzanian medicinal plant *Cussonia zimmermannii*. J Nat Prod 2007; 70(10): 1565-9. [http://dx.doi.org/10.1021/np0702133] [PMID: 17922552]

[171] Fiot J, Sanon S, Azas N, *et al.* Phytochemical and pharmacological study of roots and leaves of *Guiera senegalensis* J.F. Gmel (Combretaceae). J Ethnopharmacol 2006; 106(2): 173-8. [http://dx.doi.org/10.1016/j.jep.2005.12.030] [PMID: 16443341]

[172] Muhammad I, Li XC, Dunbar DC, ElSohly MA, Khan IA. Antimalarial (+)-tran- -hexahydrodibenzopyran derivatives from *Machaerium multiflorum*. J Nat Prod 2001; 64(10): 1322-5. [http://dx.doi.org/10.1021/np0102861] [PMID: 11678659]

[173] Vega AS, Silva Pinto AC, Nogueira KL, *et al.* Antimalarials and antioxidants compounds from *Piper tricuspe* (Piperaceae). Pharmacologyonline 2008; 1: 1-8.

[174] Tasdemir D, Brun R, Franzblau SG, Sezgin Y, Calis I. Evaluation of antiprotozoal and antimycobacterial activities of the resin glycosides and the other metabolites of *Scrophularia cryptophila*. Phytomedicine 2008; 15(3): 209-15.

CHAPTER 6

Metals as an Option for Protozoa Treatment

Norma Rivera[1], **Marcela Rojas-Lemus**[2], **Gumaro Cano-Gutierrez**[3], **Luis F. Montaño**[2] and **Teresa I. Fortoul**[2,*]

[1] *Laboratory of Malariology, Department of Microbiology and Parasitology, School of Medicine, National Autonomous University of Mexico. Mexico City, 04510, Mexico*

[2] *Department of Cellular and Tissular Biology, School of Medicine, National Autonomous University of Mexico. Mexico City, 04510, Mexico*

[3] *School of Health Sciences, UVM, Campus Sur, Mexico City, Mexico*

Abstract: Protozoa infections are a worldwide health problem that preferentially affects populations in underdeveloped countries. *Plasmodium, Leishmania, Trypanosoma, Toxoplasma, Neospora, Entamoeba* and *Trichomonas* are some of the most important genuses of protozoan parasites that infect and invade cells, tissues and organs. These parasites proliferate, migrate and mutate to evade the chemotherapeutic effects of drugs that were previously effective for their treatment. The use of metals and metals complexes to control and treat these parasites, seems a very prominent alternative. Palladium, platinum, ruthenium, antimonium, gold, iron and vanadium are some of the metals that have been evaluated as antiprotozoal treatments with favorable results. A review of the experimental effects of metal complexes on these parasites follows, along with commentary.

Keywords: Antimonium, Gold, *Leishmania*, Metal treatments, *Plasmodium*, Platinum, Palladium, Ruthenium, *Toxoplasma gondii*, *Trypanosoma*, Vanadium.

INTRODUCTION

There are 38 transition metals included in the periodic table. These metals contents ductility and malleability characteristics, frequently display numerous

* **Corresponding author Teresa I Fortoul:** Department of Cellular and Tissular Biology, School of Medicine, UNAM, Mexico City 04510, Mexico; Tel: +525556232399; Fax: 525556232182; E-mail: fortoul@unam.mx

regular oxidation states, have electrons in more than one group and are capable of conduct electricity and heat. There is a positive charge in the center of these metals that let them bind to other biomolecules of negative charge; by using these main features of the transition metals, the development of new metal-based compounds with favorable therapeutic uses, has been possible. With the discovery of cisplatin in 1965, a new field of research emerged to investigate the therapeutic features of metals [1].

The advantage in using metal based compounds instead of carbon compounds when designing new therapeutic drugs, is the ability of metals to coordinate ligands in a three dimension shape, in order to define molecular targets [2].

Treatment of protozoan experimental infections with metal compounds, are now being recognized. Protozoan parasites infect over a half billion people worldwide and continue to be one of the most significant public health problems causing a global impact. Some important human diseases caused by these pathogens include malaria, leishmaniasis, Chagas disease, toxoplasmosis, amebiasis and tri-chomoniasis. Most of the current drugs for these illnesses have been used for decades and have many limitations, such as the emergence of drug resistance, severe side-effects and low-to-medium drug efficacy; these drugs have been largely neglected as models for drug development because they are mainly used in countries with limited resources and as a consequence, with scarce marketing possibilities. Currently, there is a demand to develop new drug-based anti-protozoan therapies [3].

According to a report from the WHO, in 2013, malaria caused 584,000 deaths, with African children being the most affected population. Trypanosomiasis (sleeping sickness) has decreased in frequency, and new cases are located in Africa. From 100 to 200 new cases were reported in Chad and South Sudan in 2013. For Chagas disease, approximately 6 to 7 million people are estimated to be infected worldwide, mostly in Latin America; almost 30% of the infected people develop to a chronic phase with cardiac complications, and about 10% of these chronic patients may present digestive or neurological symptoms [4]. In addition, because the affected populations are usually located in underdeveloped countries, new treatments are not a priority for large pharmaceutical laboratories.

Leishmaniasis is distributed worldwide and is an endemic disease in more than 90 countries across almost every continent. For the treatment of leishmaniasis in humans, a selection of therapeutic compounds is offered, but the drugs are toxic and present adverse effects [5].

Worldwide, around 30% of people is infected with *Toxoplasma gondii*. Severe disease and major complications like encephalitis, myocarditis and pneumonitis are described in immunocompromised patients as a consequence of a primary infection or reactivation of a chronic one; also the fetus can be severely damage during gestation with long-term disabling sequelae, stillbirths or fetal death [6]. *Neospora caninum*, the etiologic agent of neosporosis, is an overwhelming apicomplexan parasite with worldwide distribution that causes reproductive loss in cattle and neuromuscular damage in dogs [7]. Human amebiasis caused by *E. histolytica*, is responsible for almost 50,000,000 diarrheal infections and 100,000 deaths per year. This infection is remarkably common in children from developing nations [8]. A very important sexually transmitted disease is caused by *Trichomonas vaginalis*. Trichomoniasis is a very important public health problem because it produces reproductive damage and enables the acquirement and the transmission of HIV [9].

The research of bioactive metal complexes is an opportunity to find new and less expensive treatments for these diseases [10]. This review identifies the history of these parasite infections and recollects the chemotherapy and different metals already in use along with those proposed as possible treatments for the aforementioned protozoa [11].

Table 1. Experimental use of metals against some protozoan parasites.

Parasite	***Metal/compound***	***Reference***
Leishmania	Copper	[12]
	Nickel	[13]
	Zink	[14]
	Iridium	[15]
	Palladium	[16]
	Osmium	[17]
	Vanadium	[18]

(Table 1) contd.....

Parasite	***Metal/compound***	***Reference***
Trypanosoma	Platinum (carboplatin, cisplatin, platinum with terpyridine ligands) Palladium Ruthenium Gold Rhodium Copper Osmium Vanadium	[19 - 21] [22 - 23] [24] [25] [17] [26 - 27] [28] [12] [10] [16] [27] [29] [30] [18]
Malaria	Ruthenium Gold Iron Vanadium	[28] [31] [32] [33]
Toxoplasma and Neospora	Iron Ruthenium Silver	[34] [35] [36] [37] [38] [39] [35]
Entamoeba	Ruthenium Gold Copper Manganese Iron Nikel Zinc	[27] [40] [41]
Trichomonas	Gold Palladium Iron	[42] [43] [44] [45]

Some experimental metals that have been tested under laboratory conditions against these protozoans are shown in Table **1**.

Trypanosome and Metals

The name of the disease caused by a trypanosome, Chagas, was given in honor of the man who discovered it, Carlos Ribeiro Justiniano Chagas. The disease has existed in the America for over 9,000 years, and signs of the illness were found in Peruvian mummies from which DNA samples for *T. cruzi* detection were obtained. Humans are affected by two trypanosoma species; *T. brucei* is the agent of African trypanosomiasis and is transmitted by the tse tse fly, also is known as “sleeping sickness”; T.cruzi is the etiological agent of American trypanosomiasis – Chagas disease – caused by *T. cruzi* and transmitted by the *Reduviid bugs*. Paul Ehrlich discovered in the early 20th century, the therapeutic uses of arsenophenylglycine in the treatment of African trypanosomiasis. After this finding, other metals such as sodium aurothiomalate, were evaluated to treat some diseases like kala-azar [46].

The chemotherapy for trypanosomiasis is limited. To treat the hemolymphatic stage of both West African trypanosomiasis and East African trypanosomiasis, pentamidine and suramin are the drugs of choice. Melarsoprol is used in cases of nervous system involvement. Other high toxic drugs to control African trypanosomiasis such as nitroimidazole, require around 60 days of treatment. There are studies where the activity of several metals such as gold, platinum, iridium, palladium, rhodium and osmium, were evaluated against different trypanosomatids, though their molecular targets have not been recognized [19 - 21].

Platinum complexes such as cisplatin have been used to treat this infection. Cisplatin and Carboplatin showed trypanostatic properties when tested *in vitro vs T. rhodesiensis* and, when combined with polyglutamic acid, displayed noticeable activity *in vivo* against *T. congolense* [22, 23].

Platinum complexes containing terpyridine ligands, inhibited the proliferation of *T. cruzi* amastigotes [24].

Otero *et al.* [25] reported that complexes of palladium with bioactive nitrofuran-containing thiosemicarbazones were highly active against *in vitro T. cruzi*, and the complexes were irreversible inhibitors of trypanothione reductase.

Gold complexes such like: dichloro 2- (2-pyridinyl-jN)methyl phenyl-jC Au(III); Au(III)diaceto 2- (2-pyridinyl-jN)methyl phenyl-jC-, (SP-4-3) and Au(III) 2-(mercapto-jS)benzoato(2-)-jO) 2- (2-pyridinyl-jN) methyl phenyl-jC , and the palladium complex: Aceto 2,6-bis (butylthio-jS)methyl phenyl-jC -, (SP-4- 3)-palladium(II), inhibited *T. cruzi* cathepsin B with IC_{50} values in the range of 0.2–1.4 μM and 0.4 μM, respectively [17].

Two rhenium complexes: (2(1H)-pyridinethionato-jS2) 2,6-bis (mercapto-jS)methyl)pyridine-jN1 oxorhenium(V) and chloro 2,20-(thio-jS)bis ethane-thiolato-jS) oxorhenium(V), inhibited the parasite cysteine proteases, cruzain, from *T. cruzi*. Oxorhenium compounds: ((p-methoxyphenylthiolato-S) 2,6-bis[(mercapto-jS)methyl]pyridine-jN1] oxorhenium(V) and (methanethiolato) 2,20-(thiojS) bis[ethanethiolato-jS)]] oxorhenium (V) and the palladium compound: Pd(II)aceto [2,6-bis[(butylthio-jS)methyl]phenyl-jC]-, (SP-4-3), inhibited *T. cruzi* intracellular growth. A clear structural–activity relationship was observed with the oxorhenium complexes; chloro 2,20- (thio-jS)bis[ethane-thiolato-jS)]] oxorhenium(V) was the most potent inhibitor of cathepsin B (IC_{50} of 0.009 μM) [17].

Favorable results were obtained when using ruthenium in complexes with clotrimazol and ketoconazole, these complexes, decreased the growth of *T. cruzi* epimastigotes [26 - 27]. The use of clotrimazole with ruthenium, inhibited the growth of *T. cruzi* epimastigotes in 90% [13].The activity of ketoconazole against *T. cruzi* epimastigotes was significantly improved when coordinated to ruthenium ions [12 - 13].

Coordination of clotrimazole (CTZ) with gold inhibited epimastigotes growth [47]. Coordination of CTZ to Rh, Au and Cu, affected the proliferation of *T. cruzi* epimastigotes, evaluated compounds were: RhCl(COD)(CTZ) (COD = 1,5-cyclooctadiene), AuCl3-Clotrimazole and Cu-clotrimazole [10].

Metal complexes of Mn, Fe, Co, Ni, Cu, and Zn, containing the bioactive molecule 5,7-dimethyl-1,2,4-triazolo(1,5-a)pyrimidine, were tested in *in vitro* and *in vivo* against *Trypanosoma cruzi*. All the compounds exhibited a strong extracellular and intracellular parasiticidal activity and reduced the invasion ability. The compounds showed low toxicity to macrophages and no toxicity to Vero cells [16].

Ruthenium water soluble complexes: $RuCl_2$ (HL) $(HPTA)_2$ Cl_2, with bioactive 5-nitrofuryl containing thiosemicarbazones and PTA=1,3,5-triaza-7-phosphaadamantane, were evaluated *in vitro* against *T. cruzi,*. The first complex, showed excellent parasiticidal activity with an IC_{50}=5.2 μM. The mode of action of these complexes could involve oxidative stress reactions in the parasites and could interact with DNA through an intercalative-like mode [27].

Comlpexes: cis- [RuCl(NO_2)(dppb)(5,5=-mebipy)], cis- Ru[(NO_2)2(dppb)(5,5=-mebipy)], ct-[RuCl(NO)(dppb)(5,5=-mebipy)](PF_6)$_2$, and cc-[RuCl(NO)(dppb)(5,5=-mebipy)] (PF_6)$_2$, where 5,5=-mebipy is 5,5=-dimethyl-2,2=-bipyridine and dppb is 1,4-bis(diphenylphosphino)butane, showed parasiticidal activity against *Trypanosoma cruzi*. ct- RuCl(NO) (dppb)(5,5=-mebipy) (PF_6)$_2$, diplayed a EC_{50} of 2.1-0.6 M against trypomastigotes, a IC_{50} of 1.3-0.2 M against amastigotes, and a 50% cytotoxic concentration of 51.4-0.2 M in macrophages. The nitrosyl complexes released nitric oxide into parasite, which resulted in a reduced effect of the trypanosomal protease cruzain and increased parasite autophagy and necrosis. In murine models, nitrosyl complexes reduced parasitemia and increased the survival percentage [29].

The mixed-chelate copper(II) complexes Casiopeínas® were tested *in vitro* against *T. cruzi*; its efficacy was similar to the one obtained with Nifurtimox. Casiopeínas triggered DNA cleavage through a free radical mechanism producing strong changes in tubulin, integrin and fibronectin [30].

Oxidovanadium complexes: [V^{IV}O(LASSBio1064-2H)(H_2O)], and [V^{IV}O(LASS-Bio1064-2H)(phen)](H_2O), were active *in vitro* against *T. cruzi* (Tulahuen 2 strain) epimastigotes with an IC_{50} values significantly lower than Nifurtimox. The compounds had IC_{50} > 100 mM toxicity on mammalian cells [18].

Leishmania and Metals

Leishmaniasis is caused by a variety of members from the genus *Leishmania* and is transmitted by sand flies that are usually found in desert areas. Parasites replicate inside macrophages after the infection, and infects persons while feeding. The disease has several *facades*, like cutaneous and muco-cutaneous presentations. During 1500 to 2500 BC, leishmaniasis was reported in texts that described in detail the ulcers. Kala-azar (old world visceral leishmaniasis) is characterized by fever and splenomegaly. The visceral form of the disease, is caused by *L. donovani*, *L. chagasi*, and *L. infantum*, the infection can be confused with malaria. In 1824, in Jessore, India, kala-azar was first described and misdiagnosed with malaria, but no cure was obtained using quinine, so it was suggested that it could be a different and more virulent malaria variant. Leishman and Donovan described the protozoa until the early 1900s; new species of the parasites (*L. Mexicana, L. pifanoi, L. amazonensis, L. venezuelensis* and *L. garnhami*) and some vectors, were found from Texas through Mexico, Central and South America. Clinical features were similar to those reported in Old World variants. Antimonials are the drugs of choice to treat leishmaniasis, however, resistant infections may require retreatments and the combination of Amphotericin B and ketoconazole, thus increasing toxicity in patients [16, 48].

Metal-drug synergism has been used to produce drugs by complexation of Pentamidine [13].

The combination of ruthenium ions and ketaconazole, improves the efficacy of ketoconazole against intracellular amastigotes of *L. major* [12, 13].

Copper complexes with DNA ligands such as [Cu(dppz)2]$(NO_3)_2$ have shown activity against *Leishmania braziliensis* by interacting with DNA [14].

The 4,6-dimethyl-1,2,3-triazolo[4,5-d]pyrimidin-5,7-dione, was evaluated against *L. infantum* and *L. braziliensis*; the complex was not toxic to the host cells and reduced the *in vitro* growth of amastigotes. Electron microscopy evaluation of the parasites treated with the complex, suggested organ targets such like organelle membranes [15].

Metal complexes of Mn, Fe, Co, Ni, Cu, and Zn with a bioactive molecule 5,7-dimethyl-1,2,4-triazolo[1,5-a]pyrimidine, showed an excellent parasiticidal efficacy and reduction of the invasion ability in extracellular and intracellular stages of *L. infantum* and *L. braziliensis* [16].

L. major cysteine protease (cpB) was inhibited by rhenium complexes: (2(1H)-pyridinethionato-jS2) [2,6-bis[(mercapto-jS)methyl]pyridine-jN1] oxorhenium(V) and chloro [2,20-(thio-jS)bis[(ethanethiolato-jS)]] oxorhenium(V) [17].

The palladium compound: Pd(II)aceto [2,6-bis[(butylthio-jS)methyl]phenyl-jC]-, (SP-4-3), inhibited promastigote growth in *L. major, L. mexicana, and L. donovani* [17].

Oxidovanadium complex: $[V^{IV}O(LASSBio1064\text{-}2H)(phen)](H_2O)$, showed parasiticidal activity on *L.* major promastigotes with a IC_{50} value of 22.1- 0.6 μM. The compound presented low toxicity on mammalian cells ($IC_{50} > 100$ mM), DNA could be a potential target in the parasite [18].

Plasmodium **and Metals**

Malaria is still a health problem that affects preferentially children and pregnant women [49]. From the five species that causes malaria, *P. falciparum* is the most virulent with the highest mortality rate due to nervous system involvement. The transmission vector is an *Anopheles* female mosquito with a well-known infection cycle. The problem with the disease is that the parasite has developed resistance to the few effective drugs. Here, we review some of the existing treatments and new options that include metals in their molecules. We also mention our experience with vanadium as another possible treatment. The five species that cause malaria have different distributions; *P. vivax* and *P. falciparum* are the more common species in Latin America and the Caribbean, and *P. vivax* is reported frequently in South and Central America, the Middle East and India. Worldwide, the most deadly species is *P. falciparum,* and it is usually found in Oceania, Haiti, tropical Africa, South East Asia, Dominican Republic and sections of the Amazon basin from South America. The transmission vector is a mosquito, and the season is a relevant risk factor for infection [47, 50].

The female of the infected *Anopheles* mosquito inoculates the sporozoite into the blood stream. The hepatocytes are invaded, and the production of thousands of merozoites begins rapidly. Merozoites are liberated and infect red blood cells, where their reproduction produces hemolysis; the destruction of the erythrocytes liberates merozoites that infect new hematic cells, thus concluding the asexual reproduction cycle. Few of the new expelled merozoites become gametocytes in the red cells, which evolved in gametes in the mosquito's digestive tract, and merges to result in a zygote that will become first into a motile ookinete and later into an oocyst; inside the oocyst sporozoites develop and attain the salivary glands. When an infected anopheles mosquito feeds introduces the sporozoite into the host circulation and a new cycle launches [51].

The goal of a prompt treatment for symptomatic patients aims to limit the transmission of the disease and reduce the community´s burden of malaria, which is a factor for the maintenance of the disease in the community. In the case of individuals, treatment is focused on the elimination of the asexual stages of the parasite, while at a population level, the treatments aim to limit malaria transmission and especially the transmission of drug resistant parasites [49].

Chemotherapy is the main strategy to treat malaria, and a variety of compounds have been used for this purpose, sometimes with a combination of two or three drugs reporting the best results in the treatment of the disease [50].

Treatments Against Malaria

Malaria has existed since humans and mosquitos have interacted, and symptoms have been reported since Hippocrates, describing periodic fever events in subjects that were near swamps [51, 52]. The identification of the association between the parasites and the disease occurred between the 1880-1890s; even though the understanding of the mosquito cycle developed during the 20th century helped design new approaches to control the vector, the mosquito, finding an effective treatment for prophylaxis and therapy is still a worldwide problem.

Historians have recorded that in some armed conflicts, such as the American Civil War, World War II on the Pacific coast and the Spanish-America War in 1898, casualties from malaria surpassed those that were a consequence of the armed conflicts [53].

Quinine was the first synthetic drug obtained from the cinchona bark for malaria's treatment in the first quarter of the nineteenth century, but the parasite developed resistance, and the battle against malaria experienced a setback. In some African countries, such as Zambia, malaria is killing nearly 20% of children under five years old, and the most virulent and treatment-resistant parasite is *Plasmodium falciparum.* A new threatening situation – global warming – is increasing the at risk population for infections, which is another reason to develop possible treatments against malaria [54].

Malaria has affected humankind since long ago. A cure for malaria infections has been the goal of healers and researchers for a long time, and due to diverse situations, *Plasmodium* has developed resistance to regular treatments. As we mentioned before, a variety of natural and synthetic treatments have been used, but the emerging resistance to the first option – chloroquine – has increased the interest in other options for the treatment of malaria, including the use of metals [47, 55, 56].

In Table **2** a resume of old and actual treatments for malaria is depicted.

Table 2. Traditional and new antimalarial drugs [51].

Compound	**Origin**	**Observations**	**Other relevant information**
Quinine	Chicona bark	Reported by Jesuists in Peru but for the treatment of other illness. In 1692, Richard Morton published his *Pyretologia,* mentioning its use in the treatment for "intermittent fevers". Pierre Pelletier and Joseph Caventou isolated the alkaloids quinine and cinchonine in 1820.	To reduce the bitterness of the Stem bark suspension, it was dispensed with wine.
Plasmoquine	Bayer Laboratories	In 1925 a group of chemists and biologist working together developed plasmoquine (pamaquine). This substance was the first 8-aminoquinoline proved to be useful in preventing *P. vivax* relapses.	
Mepacrine	Bayer Laboratories	Synthesized by the same group, the atebrine was use for the treatment of *P. falciparum* infection (1932).	

(Table 2) contd.....

Compound	Origin	Observations	Other relevant information
Chloroquine	Bayer Laboratories	First known as resochin, and left behind for sometime because first studies showed that it was very toxic (1934). During II World War quinine acquisition was restricted because the invasion of Java by Japan. New attempts to use the drug resurged; it was renamed as chloroquine, tested again and accepted for the treatment of malaria (1936). During 1960s resistance to chloroquine in *P. falciparum* was reported.	In 1950 Brazil introduced the use of chloroquine in cooking salt as a preventive strategy. WHO used the drug in its Global Eradication Program in the 1950s and 1960s. At the same time DDT was used to eradicate the vector.
Pyrimethamine	Burroughs-Wellcome Laboratories	Resulted from proguanil, developed by the British scientist during World War II.	Pyrimethamine
Atovaquone	Glaxo-Wellcome Pharmaceutics	Derived from 2-hydroxynaphtoquinones during World War II.	Atovaquone
Artemisinin (qinghao)	Artemisia annua	Used in Chinese herbal remedies, for the treatment of hemorrhoids for at least 2000 years. Li Shizhen in 1596 suggested its use in the treatment of fever in a cold-water extract. As an effort to explore the utility of old herbal remedies, the government of the People's Republic of China in 1972 explored qinghao, and the active ingredient was purified, and tested in patients with promising results that were published in early 1980s.	Artemisinin (qinghao)

Promising possibilities are emerging for metals in complex with other compounds; examples include those for which resistance has developed and those used as treatments for other parasites, such as *T. cruzi* and *Leishmania* have shown its effectiveness [57]. In our laboratory, CD-1 mice infected with *P. yoelii yoelii* were exposed to vanadium inhalation [58], and in preliminary results after a three-day exposure, the exposed mice showed a drastic decrease in parasitemia, malaria pigment and an increased survival compared with infected controls that had 100% mortality [59].

The coordination of CQ to ruthenium in the complex $RuCl_2(CQ)_2$ was effective to circumvent the resistance mechanism in the case of *P. falciparum* during *in vivo* tests (*P. berghei*). The Ru complex reduced parasitemia in 94% of the treated groups [28].

In *in vitro* experiments, the complex $(Au(CQ)(PPh_3))[PF_6]$ was active against the chloroquine-resistant FcB1 strain of *Plasmodium falciparum* and against the rodent malarial parasite *P. berghei* [31].

The ferrocenyl moiety, linked to a side chain of a 4-aminoquinoline, resulted in a potent chloroquine analog called ferroquine, which was active against *P. falciparum* chloroquine-resistant strains. FQ also exhibited remarkably high antimalarial activity *in vivo* in mice infected with *Plasmodium berghei*, *Plasmodium yoelii* and *Plasmodium vinckei vinckei* [32].

The gold(I) complex $Au(CQ)(PPh_3)$ NO_3 was effective against W2 and K1 *P. falciparum* strains; $Au(CQ)(PMe_3)$ $[PF_6]$ and $Au(CQ)(PEt_3)$ $[PF_6]$ were active against the FcB1 *P. falciparum* strain [34]. Other reports regarding the evaluation of antimalarial activity for gold complexes against chloroquine-sensitive and chloroquine-resistant strains of *Plasmodium* parasites are compiled in an excellent review by Glišić and Djuran [60].

In Table **3**, some metals for the treatment of *Trypanosoma*, *Leishmania* and malaria are shown.

Table 3. Metal complexes as chemotherapeutic agents against *Leishmania, Trypanosoma* and malaria.

Compound	**Origin**	**Observations**
Heteroleptic oxivanadium(iv) compounds [56].	Facultad de Química UDELAR, Montevideo Uruguay	These compounds have not been tested in the treatment of malaria, but because its promising effectiveness in Trypanosomiasis, these bioactive vanadium compounds emerge as a possibility.
Water-soluble Ruthenium Complexes [27].	Facultad de Química, DEC, UDELAR, Montevideo, Uruguay	Ruthenium complexes were proved against *T. cruzi* and *E. histolyticain vitro* with promising results. Also a promising option in the treatment of malaria.

(Table 3) contd.....

Compound	Origin	Observations
Metallodrugs such as: auranofin, aurothiomalate, triethylphosphinegold(I) chloride, cysplatin, ruthenium(III) complex NAMI-A, mononuclear and dinuclear gold(III) complexes, bismuth and antimony compounds [57].	Department of Pharmacokinetics. University of Groningen, The Netherlands	Different compounds are been tested as possible treatments against malaria; at least *in vitro* reduce the growth of *P. falciparum*.
Different Gold complexes are being tested as potential antimalarial agents and for the treatment of tripanosomiasis [47].	Lab. Química Bioinorgánica, IVIC, Caracas, Venezuela.	Attaching Gold to Chloroquine has reported to be active against two resistant strains of *P. falciparum* as well as Gold (III) complexes. Auranofin inhibits the growth of *P. falciparum*. Usually when coordinated with clotrimazol the inhibition of epmastigotes of *T. cruzi* increases.
Inhaled Vanadium pentoxide eliminates the parasitemia and the haem pigment, increasing mice survival.	Cellular and Tissular Biology Department and Malariology Laboratory, Dept. Microbiology and Parasitology. School of Medicine, UNAM	CD-1 male mice infected with *P.yoelii yoelii* were exposed twice a week for one week to vanadium pentoxide and a notorious decrease in parasitemia was observed in exposed mice compared with controls. Also survival increased in exposed mice.
Antimonials alone or in combination with amphotericin B and pentamidin Zinc sulphate Selenium Peroxovanadium compounds [16].	School of Chemistry, University of Birmingham, UK Dept. Inorganic Chemistry School of Sciences, Univ. Granada Spain Dept. Parasitology, School of Sciences, Univ. Granada, Spain.	Antimonials for the treatment of Leishmania Zinc sulphate for the treatment of *L.major* and *L. tropica*. Selenium with Vitamin E for the treatment of *T. cruzi* Peroxovanadium compounds in the treatment of Leishmania
Palladium and Platinum complexes with 5-nitrofuryl-containing thiosemicarbazones [26].	Cátedra de Química Orgánica, U de la R, Gral Flores, Montevideo, Uruguay	Its main actions were on *T. cruzi*
Palladium complexes with bioactive nitrofuran-containing thiosemicarbazones [25].	Cátedra de Química Inorgánica, Dept. Estrella Campos, Facultad de Química, Universidad de la República, Montevideo, Uruguay	*In vitro* the complexes were highly active against *T. cruzi* compared with Nifurtimox. The complexes were irreversible inhibitors of trypanothione reductase.

Toxoplasma, Neospora and Metals

Toxoplasma gondii and *Neospora caninum* are both apicomplexan parasites with worldwide distribution. *T. gondii* is a parasite of both human and veterinary interest that may cause serious pathology in immune-compromised individuals and has produced high economic impact in livestock, especially in sheep. *N. caninum* represents one of the most important infectious causes of bovine abortion with an economic impact and causes neuromuscular disease in dogs [61]. An important feature of these apicomplexa is that they are able to invade and replicate within a wide range of nucleated cells inside a parasitophorous vacuole. Repeated cycles of schizogony replication including invasion, proliferation, and egress of tachyzoites, are responsible for inducing acute toxoplasmosis and the pathological damage that occur during the acute infection. After some schizogony replications, chronic toxoplasmosis takes place with the conversion from tachyzoites into bradyzoites, and the development of intracellular tissue cysts in different organs and tissues like brain, and skeletal muscles [62].

The ubiquity existence of *Toxoplasma gondii*, the lack of drugs to kill tissue cysts, the current use of a treatment with several side effects, and the absence of commercial vaccines, highlight the urgent need to develop new drugs with high efficacy against *T. gondii*. Currently, there are no efficient treatments available to eliminate all forms of *Toxoplasma* in the host [39]. Bradyzoites and tissue cysts are infective forms that cannot be easily destroyed by conventional anti-toxoplasmic treatments. Compounds that have been used in toxoplasmosis treatment include sulfonamides, clindamycin, macrolides and hydroxy-naphthoquinones. All these agents show clear effects against the viability of extracellular tachyzoites; however they have limited or null activity toward intracellular parasites located within PVs or on tissue cysts.

The effect of bovine Lactoferrin (bLf) in its nanoformulation (AEC-CCo-CP--Lf-NC) was analyzed against *T. gondii. In vitro* analysis showed an increase in nitric oxide production and low parasitemia. *In vivo* analysis of BALB/c mice showed an increased level of reactive oxygen species, nitric oxide production, and Th1 cytokine, which helped in parasite clearance. The parasite load in various organs decreased and aided in the survival of mice until day 25 post-infection.

The mechanism of action for the nanoformulation, clarified by immunoreactivity, showed accumulation of Lf in macrophages of various visceral organs, which is the site of parasite multiplication [34].

Two hydrolytically stable ruthenium complexes, were tested against *T. gondii* and *N. caninum* and exhibited 50% inhibitory concentrations of 18.7 and 41.1 nM in the first parasite and 6.7 and 11.3 nM in the second one. Transmission electron microscopy showed ultrastructural changes in both parasites [35].

Silver nanoparticles demonstrated highly toxoplasmicidal activity when used singly or in combination with chitosan. When tested *in vivo*, the mean percentage of thacyzoites purified from the liver and spleen, decreased in an evident number and the parasites showed evident changes in their shape [36].

Due to the increasing importance of the role of Fe in intracellular proliferation for *Toxoplasma*, various strategies have been designed to limit parasite development by using Fe chelating agents, such as desferrioxamine. In studies of *Toxoplasma* invasion and proliferation in primary cultures of rat enterocytes (cells that form part of the intestine epithelium), exposure to desferrioxamine inhibited the intracellular replication of tachyzoites and was considered a promising drug against acute toxoplasmosis in mice, prolonging mice survival [37].

Exposure of *T. gondii* tachyzoites to Lactoferricin (Lfcin), a peptide composed of 25 amino acids formed by pepsin, has harmful effects on parasites, decreasing their invasive capability in embryonic rat cells. Similarly, mice previously treated with Lfcin showed a higher survival index after intraperitoneal inoculation of *Toxoplasma* tachyzoites. The effect of Lfcin (0.5-5.0 mg/ml) has been evaluated in brain rat cysts obtained from the Berverley strain of *T. gondii*. Oral administration of Lfcin in infected animals showed a protective function dependent on the doses. It is thought that Lfcin binds to the parasite membrane, destroying the pellicle and decreasing the infective capability [38].

The anti-Toxoplasma activity of the compound [Fe (HPClNOL) (SO_4)]2-μ-oxo, significantly reduced the level of parasite infection in host cells, leading to a severe reduction of the parasite antioxidant enzymes superoxide dismutase and catalase as a consequence of the induction of reactive oxygen species by the compound [39].

Ruthenium-based compounds containing heteroatom ligands like azole derivatives, and NAMI-A and KP-1019, completely inhibited the proliferation of both *T. gondii* and *N. caninum,* with *N. caninum* being more susceptible [35].

Entamoeba histolytica and Metals

Novel ruthenium water soluble complexes like $RuCl_2(HL)(HPTA)_2\ Cl_2$, with HL =bioactive 5-nitrofuryl containing thiosemicarbazones and PTA=1,3,5-triaza-7-phosphaadamantane, showed excellent activity against *Entamoeba histolytica* with a half maximal inhibitory concentration (IC_{50})=5.2 µM. It seems that the mechanisms of action of these compounds, involved oxidative interactions with DNA [27].

The complexes $Au(PPh_3)(1)\ PF_6$ (2), $Ru(1)2(Cl)_2(H_2O)_2$ (3), and Cu(1)2 (_-Cl)(H_2O) $2Cl_2$ (4), were evaluated *in vitro* as against *Entamoeba histolytica* HM1: IMSS strain. Their IC_{50} values were in the range of 0.10 ± 0.51 (Table **2**), which makes these drugs, considerably more potent than the uncomplexed metronidazole [40].

The N6 ligand 2,9-bis-(2′,5′-diazahexanyl)-1,10-phenanthroline (L1) and the corresponding coordination compounds of L1, with the divalent cations of essential metals Mn, Fe, Co, Ni, Cu and Zn, were tested against axenic cultures *Entamoeba histolytica* (HM1:IMSS strain). The compounds with Ni and Mn presented the best amoebicide activities with IC_{50} values of 60 nM and 80 nM, respectively [41].

Trichomonas vaginalis and Metals

Pd(II) complexes containing salicylaldiminato thiosemicarbazones as dinegative tridentate ligands were tested *in vitro* against *Trichomonas vaginalis* parasite, exhibiting a percentage of inhibition greater than 80 at 100 µM [42].

The gold complexes 1,2-bis(diphenylphosphino)ethane-bis-(gold(I)- lupinylsulfi-dehydrochloride) and triethylphosphinogold(I)-(2-diethylamino) ethylsulfi-dehydrochloride were evaluated *in vitro* against *Trichomonas vaginalis* OZ-2, isolated from a case of vaginal trichomoniasis [43].

Lactoferrin has showed to specifically binds to surface receptors of *Trichomonas* and it concentrates in specific places of the infected mucosa; so, these features makes lactoferrin a possible carrier for drugs delivery [44].

According to Alvarez-Sánchez *et al.* 2007, iron specifically down-regulates proteolytic activity, expression, and transcription of CP65, negatively affecting *Trichomonas vaginalis* cytotoxicity *in vitro* [45].

CONCLUSION

The treatment options for protozoan diseases have increased, with the regular chemotherapeutic options being expanded to include complexes of metals, including drugs with reported resistance from the protozoa. Several groups are working on different metals, and promising results are emerging. More studies with an increased variety of metals will provide possibility to obtain cheaper and more effective treatments for populations in underdeveloped countries; thus, more work must be performed to discover metal compounds that are more selective in interacting with therapeutic targets.

CONFLICT OF INTEREST

The authors confirm that they have no conflict of interest to declare for this publication.

ACKNOWLEDGEMENTS

The authors are grateful to the project: PAPIIT-DGAPA UNAM IA203015.

GLOSSARY

Apicomplexa = A phylum of obligate intracellular parasites which possess common structures in their apical complex like spirally arranged microtubules, rhoptries, micronemes and dense granules, that help the parasites into the invasion and replication cycle. Some examples of this phylum are Malaria, *Toxplasma gondii* , *Neospora caninum* , *Cryptosporidium* spp.

Bradyzoites = *Toxoplasma gondii* intracellular parasite stage of slow replication. They convert the host cell into a tissue cyst.

Lactoferrin = Is a glycoprotein located in the secretions from exocrine glands and neutrophils granules. This protein possesses antimicrobial properties and iron binding ability.

Malaria pigment = During the digestion of hemoglobin by *Plasmodium* spp parasites, high quantities of free heme are released, the parasites have to convert this toxic heme into insoluble hemozoin that is named malaria pigment.

Merozoite = Stage parasite that is released after a schizogony, these parasites can start a new sexual or asexual cycle.

Metal complexes = Complexes that consists of a metallic central atom, surrounded by an array of molecules.

Ookinete = Parasite stage in the mosquito´s body that develops into an oocyst and is formed by the fertilization of both macrogametes and microgametes.

Palladium = Transition metal included in the group of the platinum metals (iridium, osmium, platinum, rhodium and ruthenium). They are resistant to chemical attack and have stable electrical properties.

Parasitophorous vacuole = Intracellular structure formed by apicomplexan parasites that allows them to developed in a safe environment.

Vanadium = Is a transition metal with lithophile and siderophile features. Is a highly mobile element that can be found in the soil, water and air and in living organisms.

Schizogony = The asexual reproduction of the sporozoite parasite stage that forms new merozoites.

Sporozoite = Infective intracellular parasite stages that are released by the oocyst of the apicomplexan parasites.

Tachyzoites = *Toxoplasma gondii* intracellular parasite stage of rapid replication and the cause of acute toxoplasmosis.

REFERENCES

[1] Rafique S, Idrees M, Nasim A, Akbar H, Athar A. Transition metal complexes as potential therapeutic agents. Biotech Mol Biol Rev 2010; 5(2): 38-45.

[2] Frezza M, Hindo S, Chen D, *et al.* Novel metals and metal complexes as platforms for cancer therapy. Curr Pharm Des 2010; 16(16): 1813-25.
[PMID: 20337575]

[3] Martins Alho MA, Marrero-Ponce Y, Barigye SJ, *et al.* Antiprotozoan lead discovery by aligning dry and wet screening: prediction, synthesis, and biological assay of novel quinoxalinones. Bioorg Med Chem 2014; 22(5): 1568-85.
[PMID: 24513185]

[4] World Health Organization [homepage on the internet]. cWHO, 2015 Health topics" [cited 12th November 2015]. Available from: http://www.who.int/topics/en/.

[5] Barbosa JF, de Figueiredo SM, Monteiro FM, *et al.* New approaches on leishmaniasis treatment and prevention: a review of recent patents. Recent Pat Endocr Metab Immune Drug Discov 2015; 9(2): 90-102.
[PMID: 26392062]

[6] Liu Q, Wang Z-D, Huang S-Y, Zhu X-Q. Diagnosis of toxoplasmosis and typing of *Toxoplasma gondii.* Parasit Vectors 2015; 8: 292.
[PMID: 26017718]

[7] Donahoe SL, Lindsay SA, Krockenberger M, Phalen D, Šlapeta J. A review of neosporosis and pathologic findings of *Neospora caninum* infection in wildlife. Int J Parasitol Parasites Wildl 2015; 4(2): 216-38.
[PMID: 25973393]

[8] Ralston KS. Taking a bite: Amoebic trogocytosis in *Entamoeba histolytica* and beyond. Curr Opin Microbiol 2015; 28(28): 26-35.
[PMID: 26277085]

[9] Kissinger P. Trichomonas vaginalis: a review of epidemiologic, clinical and treatment issues. BMC Infect Dis 2015; 15(15): 307.
[PMID: 26242185]

[10] Sánchez-Delgado RA, Anzellotti A, Suárez L. Metal complexes as chemotherapeutic agents against tropical diseases: malaria, *trypanosomiasis*, and *leishmaniasis*. Met Ions Biol Syst 2004; 41: 379-419.
[PMID: 15206123]

[11] Swann J, Jamshidi N, Lewis NE, Winzeler EA. Systems analysis of host-parasite interactions. Wiley Interdiscip Rev Syst Biol Med 2015; 7(6): 381-400.
[PMID: 26306749]

[12] Iniguez E, Sánchez A, Vasquez MA, *et al.* Metal-drug synergy: new ruthenium(II) complexes of ketoconazole are highly active against Leishmania major and Trypanosoma cruzi and nontoxic to human or murine normal cells. J Biol Inorg Chem 2013; 18(7): 779-90.
[PMID: 23881220]

[13] Sánchez-Delgado RA, Lazardi K, Rincón L, Urbina JA. Toward a novel metal-based chemotherapy against tropical diseases. 1. Enhancement of the efficacy of clotrimazole against *Trypanosoma cruzi* by complexation to ruthenium in RuCl2(clotrimazole)2. J Med Chem 1993; 36(14): 2041-3.
[PMID: 8336342]

[14] Navarro M, Cisneros-Fajardo EJ, Sierralta A, *et al.* Design of copper DNA intercalators with leishmanicidal activity. J Biol Inorg Chem 2003; 8(4): 401-8.
[PMID: 12761661]

[15] Ramírez-Macías I, Maldonado CR, Marín C, *et al. In vitro* anti-leishmania evaluation of nickel complexes with a triazolopyrimidine derivative against *Leishmania infantum* and *Leishmania braziliensis*. J Inorg Biochem 2012; 112: 1-9.
[PMID: 22542591]

[16] Caballero AB, Rodríguez-Diéguez A, Quirós M, *et al.* Triazolopyrimidine compounds containing first-row transition metals and their activity against the neglected infectious Chagas disease and leishmaniasis. Eur J Med Chem 2014; 85: 526-34.
[PMID: 25127147]

[17] Fricker SP, Mosi RM, Cameron BR, *et al.* Metal compounds for the treatment of parasitic diseases. J Inorg Biochem 2008; 102(10): 1839-45.

[PMID: 18684510]

[18] Benítez J, Cavalcanti de Queiroz A, Correia I, *et al.* New oxidovanadium(IV) N-acylhydrazone complexes: promising antileishmanial and antitrypanosomal agents. Eur J Med Chem 2013; 62: 20-7. [PMID: 23353731]

[19] Croft SL, Neal RA, Craciunescu DG, Certad-Fombona G. The activity of platinum, iridium and rhodium drug complexes against *Leishmania donovani.* Trop Med Parasitol 1992; 43(1): 24-8. [PMID: 1598504]

[20] Loiseau PM, Craciunescu DG, Doadrio-Villarejo JC, Certad-Fombona G, Gayral P. Pharmacomodulations on new organometallic complexes of Ir, Pt, Rh, Pd, Os: *in vitro* and *in vivo* trypanocidal study against *Trypanosoma brucei brucei.* Trop Med Parasitol 1992; 43(2): 110-4. [PMID: 1519021]

[21] Rodriguez-Cabezas MN, Mesa-Valle CM, Azzouz S, *et al. In vitro* and *in vivo* activity of new rhodium (III) complexes against *Leishmania donovani.* Pharmacology 2001; 63(2): 112-9. [PMID: 11490204]

[22] Farrell NP. Transition Metal Complexes as Drugs and Chemotherapeutic Agents. Springer Science & Business Media. 1989; 11: pp. 222-42.

[23] Kinnamon KE, Steck EA, Rane DS. Activity of antitumor drugs against African trypanosomes. Antimicrob Agents Chemother 1979; 15(2): 157-60. [PMID: 426509]

[24] Bonse S, Richards JM, Ross SA, Lowe G, Krauth-Siegel RL. (2, 2': 6', 2''-Terpyridine) platinum (II) Complexes Are Irreversible Inhibitors of *Trypanosoma* c ruzi *Trypanothione Reductase* But Not of Human Glutathione Reductase. J Med Chem 2000; 43(25): 4812-21.

[25] Otero L, Vieites M, Boiani L, *et al.* Novel antitrypanosomal agents based on palladium nitrofurylthiosemicarbazone complexes: DNA and redox metabolism as potential therapeutic targets. J Med Chem 2006; 49(11): 3322-31. [PMID: 16722651]

[26] Cipriani M, Toloza J, Bradford L, *et al.* Effect of the Metal Ion on the anti T. cruzi Activity and Mechanism of Action of 5-Nitrofuryl-Containing Thiosemicarbazone Metal Complexes. Eur J Inorg Chem 2014; 27: 4677-89.

[27] Sarniguet C, Toloza J, Cipriani M, *et al.* Water-soluble ruthenium complexes bearing activity against protozoan parasites. Biol Trace Elem Res 2014; 159(1-3): 379-92. [PMID: 24740394]

[28] Sánchez-Delgado RA, Navarro M, Pérez H, Urbina JA. Toward a novel metal-based chemotherapy against tropical diseases. 2. Synthesis and antimalarial activity *in vitro* and *in vivo* of new ruthenium- and rhodium-chloroquine complexes. J Med Chem 1996; 39(5): 1095-9. [PMID: 8676344]

[29] Bastos TM, Barbosa MI, da Silva MM, *et al.* Nitro/nitrosyl-ruthenium complexes are potent and selective anti-*Trypanosoma cruzi* agents causing autophagy and necrotic parasite death. Antimicrob Agents Chemother 2014; 58(10): 6044-55. [PMID: 25092707]

[30] Becco L, Rodríguez A, Bravo ME, *et al.* New achievements on biological aspects of copper complexes Casiopeínas®: interaction with DNA and proteins and anti-Trypanosoma cruzi activity. J Inorg Biochem 2012; 109: 49-56.
[PMID: 22377716]

[31] Navarro M, Pérez H, Sánchez-Delgado RA. Toward a novel metal-based chemotherapy against tropical diseases. 3. Synthesis and antimalarial activity *in vitro* and *in vivo* of the new gold-chloroquine complex [Au(PPh3)(CQ)]PF6. J Med Chem 1997; 40(12): 1937-9.
[PMID: 9191972]

[32] Biot C, Glorian G, Maciejewski LA, Brocard JS. Synthesis and antimalarial activity *in vitro* and *in vivo* of a new ferrocene-chloroquine analogue. J Med Chem 1997; 40(23): 3715-8.
[PMID: 9371235]

[33] Navarro M, Vásquez F, Sánchez-Delgado RA, Pérez H, Sinou V, Schrével J. Toward a novel metal-based chemotherapy against tropical diseases. 7. Synthesis and *in vitro* antimalarial activity of new gold-chloroquine complexes. J Med Chem 2004; 47(21): 5204-9.
[PMID: 15456263]

[34] Anand N, Sehgal R, Kanwar RK, Dubey ML, Vasishta RK, Kanwar JR. Oral administration of encapsulated bovine lactoferrin protein nanocapsules against intracellular parasite *Toxoplasma gondii.* Int J Nanomedicine 2015; 10: 6355-69.
[PMID: 26504384]

[35] Barna F, Debache K, Vock CA, Küster T, Hemphill A. *In vitro* effects of novel ruthenium complexes in *Neospora caninum* and *Toxoplasma gondii* tachyzoites. Antimicrob Agents Chemother 2013; 57(11): 5747-54.
[PMID: 23979747]

[36] Gaafar MR, Mady RF, Diab RG, Shalaby TI. Chitosan and silver nanoparticles: promising anti-toxoplasma agents. Exp Parasitol 2014; 143: 30-8.
[PMID: 24852215]

[37] Mahmoud MS. Effect of deferoxamine alone and combined with pyrimethamine on acute toxoplasmosis in mice. J Egypt Soc Parasitol 1999; 29(3): 791-803.
[PMID: 12561919]

[38] Isamida T, Tanaka T, Omata Y, Yamauchi K, Shimazaki K, Saito A. Protective effect of lactoferricin against *Toxoplasma gondii* infection in mice. J Vet Med Sci 1998; 60(2): 241-4.
[PMID: 9524950]

[39] Portes JA, Souza TG, dos Santos TA, *et al.* Reduction of *Toxoplasma gondii* development due to inhibition of parasite antioxidant enzymes by a dinuclear iron(III) compound. Antimicrob Agents Chemother 2015; 59(12): 7374-86.
[PMID: 26392498]

[40] Athar F, Husain K, Abid M, *et al.* Synthesis and anti-amoebic activity of gold(I), ruthenium(II), and copper(II) complexes of metronidazole. Chem Biodivers 2005; 2(10): 1320-30.
[PMID: 17191933]

[41] García-Ramos JC, Toledano-Magaña Y, Talavera-Contreras LG, *et al.* Potential cytotoxic and

amoebicide activity of first row transition metal compounds with 2,9-bis-(2′,5′-diazahexanyl)-1,1-phenanthroline (L1). Dalton Trans 2012; 41(34): 10164-74.
[PMID: 22722265]

[42] Chellan P, Stringer T, Shokar A, *et al.* Synthesis and *in vitro* evaluation of palladium(II) salicylaldiminato thiosemicarbazone complexes against Trichomonas vaginalis. J Inorg Biochem 2011; 105(12): 1562-8.
[PMID: 22071079]

[43] Novelli F, Recine M, Sparatore F, Juliano C. Gold(I) complexes as antimicrobial agents. Farmaco 1999; 54(4): 232-6.
[PMID: 10384716]

[44] Sehgal R, Goyal K, Sehgal A. Trichomoniasis and lactoferrin: future prospects Infect Dis Obstet Gynecol 2012; 2012; 536037.

[45] Alvarez-Sánchez ME, Solano-González E, Yañez-Gómez C, Arroyo R. Negative iron regulation of the CP65 cysteine proteinase cytotoxicity in Trichomonas vaginalis. Microbes Infect 2007; 9(14-15): 1597-605.
[PMID: 18023389]

[46] Caballero AB, Salas JM, Sánchez-Moreno M. Metal-Based Therapeutics for Leishmaniasis. In: David M Claborn, Ed. Chapter 20 Leishmaniasis - Trends in Epidemiology, Diagnosis and Treatment. Intech [E-book]. Published: March 19, 2014. Available from: http://www.intechopen.com/books/leishmaniasis-trends-in-epidemiology-diagnosis-and-treatment/metal-based-therape-tics-for-leishmaniasis

[47] Navarro M. Gold complexes as potential anti-parasitic agents. Coord Chem Rev 2009; 253: 1619-26.

[48] Ridley JW. Blood (intracellular) and other tissue protozoa. In: Ridley JW, Ed. Parasitology for medical and clinical Laboratory professionals. New York: DELMAR CENGAGE Learning 2012.

[49] Bardach A, Ciapponi A, Rey-Ares L, *et al.* Epidemiology of Malaria in Latin America and the Caribbean from 1990 to 2009: Systematic Review and Meta-Analysis. Value in Health Regional Issues 2015; 8: 69-79.

[50] Navarro M, Gabbiani C, Messori L, Gambino D. Metal-based drugs for malaria, trypanosomiasis and leishmaniasis: recent achievements and perspectives. Drug Discov Today 2010; 15(23-24): 1070-8.
[PMID: 20974285]

[51] Barnes KI. Antimalarial Drugs and the Control and Elimination of Malaria. In: Sataines HM, Krishna S, Ed. Treatment and prevention of Malaria: Springer Basel AG. 2012; pp. 1-17.

[52] Meshnick S, Dobson MJ. The history of antimalarial drugs. In: Rosenthal PJ, Ed. Antimalarial chemotherapy. New Jersey: Humana Press. 2001; pp. 15-25.

[53] Finkel M. Stoping a global killer: Malaria Nat Geo Magazine July 2007. [cited:12th Nov 2015]; [15p]. Available from: http://ngm.nationalgeographic.com/2007/07/malaria/finkel-text

[54] Garcia LS. Malaria. Clin Lab Med 2010; 30(1): 93-129.
[PMID: 20513543]

[55] Mesa-Valle CM, Rodriguez-Cabezas MN, Moraleda-Lindez V, Craciunescu D, Sanchez-Moreno M, Osuna A. *In vitro* and *in vivo* activity of two Pt(IV) salts against leishmania donovani. Pharmacology

1998; 57(3): 160-72.
[PMID: 9691236]

[56] Fernández M, Varela J, Correia I, *et al.* A new series of heteroleptic oxidovanadium(IV) compounds with phenanthroline-derived co-ligands: selective *Trypanosoma cruzi* growth inhibitors. Dalton Trans 2013; 42(33): 11900-11.
[PMID: 23787783]

[57] Almeida A, Oliviera BL, Correia J, Soveral G, Casini A. Emerging protein targets for metal-based pharmaceutical agents: An update. Coord Chem Rev 2013; 257: 2689-704.

[58] Fortoul TI, González-Villalva A, Rojas-Lemus M, *et al.* Inhalation of vanadium pentoxide and its toxic effects in a mouse model. Inorg Chim Acta 2014; 420: 8-15.

[59] Rivera Fernández N, Colín Barenque L, Romero Silva SE, *et al.* Ependymal damage in a Plasmodium yoelii yoelii lethal murine malaria model. Histol Histopathol 2015; 30(2): 245-53.
[PMID: 25252586]

[60] Glišić BĐ, Djuran MI. Gold complexes as antimicrobial agents: an overview of different biological activities in relation to the oxidation state of the gold ion and the ligand structure. Dalton Trans 2014; 43(16): 5950-69.
[PMID: 24598838]

[61] Dubey JP, Schares G, Ortega-Mora LM. Epidemiology and control of neosporosis and Neospora caninum. Clin Microbiol Rev 2007; 20(2): 323-67.
[PMID: 17428888]

[62] Winzer P, Müller J, Aguado-Martínez A, *et al.* *In Vitro* and *In Vivo* Effects of the Bumped Kinase Inhibitor 1294 in the Related Cyst-Forming Apicomplexans *Toxoplasma gondii* and *Neospora caninum*. Antimicrob Agents Chemother 2015; 59(10): 6361-74.
[PMID: 26248379]

SUBJECT INDEX

D

K

L

M

N

O

P

Made in United States
Orlando, FL
04 November 2026

90207784R00116